PRAISE FOR ROGER FRE

THE FLEXIBLE G

"I AM VERY PLEASED TO SEE THAT ROGER IS NOW BRINGING THE PRINCIPLES OF ANATOMICAL FUNCTION INTO THE GOLF WORLD, WHERE I BELIEVE THAT THEY WILL HAVE A SUBSTANTIAL IMPACT ON NOT ONLY YOUR GOLF SWING, BUT ALSO CARRY OVER INTO YOUR EVERYDAY LIFE AS WELL."

—JACK NICKLAUS, MEMBER, WORLD GOLF HALL OF FAME

"ROGER AND I ADAMANTLY BELIEVE THAT IN ORDER TO PLAY GREAT GOLF ONE HAS TO BE FLEXIBLE, STRONG, AND EAT CORRECTLY. IF YOU WANT A BETTER GOLF GAME, ROGER'S THE MAN TO HELP YOU."

—GARY PLAYER, MEMBER, WORLD GOLF HALL OF FAME

"TODAY THERE IS MORE UNDERSTANDING OF THE RELATIONSHIP BETWEEN BEING FIT AND PLAYING GOOD GOLF. IT IS DIFFICULT TO HAVE ONE WITHOUT THE OTHER. ROGER'S INSTRUCTION AND STRETCHING EXERCISES WILL NO DOUBT ACCELERATE YOUR PATH FROM WANTING TO BE A GOOD PLAYER TO ACTUALLY BECOMING ONE."

—TOM KITE, MEMBER, WORLD GOLF HALL OF FAME

"I HONESTLY BELIEVE THAT ROGER'S PROGRAM IS THE BEST THAT I'VE EVER SEEN FOR AMATEURS OR PROS."

—DONNA CAPONI, MEMBER, WORLD GOLF HALL OF FAME

"ROGER'S PROGRAM WILL HELP YOU ON AND OFF THE COURSE, JUST LIKE IT DID FOR ME."

—BERNHARD LANGER, MEMBER, WORLD GOLF HALL OF FAME

"IN THIS BOOK, ROGER REVEALS THE 'SECRETS' TO THE GAME OF GOLF. HE HAS DONE A GREAT JOB EXPLAINING HOW YOUR BODY DICTATES YOUR PERFORMANCE, HOW GOLF (LIKE ALL SPORTS) REQUIRES BALANCE, AND HOW A FUNCTIONAL BODY IS THE KEY TO EXECUTING A FUNDAMENTAL GOLF SWING."

—PETE EGOSCUE, FOUNDER OF THE EGOSCUE METHOD; AUTHOR OF THE *PAIN FREE* BOOK SERIES

"ROGER'S PROGRAM IS THE BEST. IF HE CAN TAKE AN OLD GUY LIKE ME AND MAKE ME WIN THE SENIOR PGA AT 58, I'LL TELL YOU WHAT, HIS PROGRAM MUST WORK!"

—JOHN "J. J." JACOBS, 2003 SENIOR PGA CHAMPION

THE
FLEXIBLE
GOLF SWING

THE
FLEXIBLE
GOLF SWING

A CUTTING-EDGE GUIDE TO IMPROVING FLEXIBILITY
AND MASTERING GOLF'S TRUE FUNDAMENTALS

ROGER FREDERICKS
FOREWORD BY ARNOLD PALMER

RODALE.

© 2010, 2014 by Roger Fredericks

Photos courtesy of the author except: Images for Figs. 2.5, 2.6 & 3.28 © Getty Images; Fig. 2.10 © erikdalton.com

Rodale books may be purchased for business or promotional use or for special sales. For information, please write to: Special Markets Department, Rodale Inc., 733 Third Avenue, New York, NY 10017

Printed in the United States of America
Rodale Inc. makes every effort to use acid-free ♾, recycled paper ♻.

Book design by Christopher Rhoads

Library of Congress Cataloging-in-Publication Data is on file with the publisher.

ISBN 978–1–62336–139–6   paperback

Distributed to the trade by Macmillan

2   4   6   8   10   9   7   5   3   1   paperback

We inspire and enable people to improve their lives and the world around them.
rodalebooks.com

*This book is dedicated to my father, the late Elmer Fredericks,
for introducing me to the greatest game the world has ever known,
which has taught me that golf is much more than a game.*

CONTENTS

FOREWORD

EARLY IN THE WEEK at the 2003 Senior PGA Championship at Aronimink Golf Club, in Newtown Square, Pennsylvania, I played a practice round with my longtime friend and fellow Tour professional Tommy Jacobs.

I hadn't played with Tommy for a number of years, but the thing that caught my attention was how far he was hitting his drives. At the time, he was close to 70 years old, and he was bombing the ball—he was as long as most pros who are 20 years younger. I told Tommy how surprised I was that he hadn't lost any distance, like the rest of us had.

Tommy informed me that he had actually *gained* a lot of distance because he had embarked on a unique flexibility program developed by a PGA professional and fitness expert named Roger Fredericks.

For the next year, it seemed like everywhere I went, Roger's name kept popping up in conversations, as more and more friends and golf professionals had caught wind of his program, and they too were giving testimonials to the great results that his program had given them.

Finally, in December of 2004, I was introduced to Roger by my friend David Chapman at a course that I had designed, the Tradition Golf Club in La Quinta, California.

Roger had put together videos of my current golf swing and compared them to my swing as a younger man. Then he ran me through some simple but very revealing flexibility tests, in which, I must admit, I performed poorly. At that point, Roger explained precisely how my lack of flexibility as demonstrated by these tests had directly contributed to the restrictions that we had just seen in my golf swing. He explained to me, in no uncertain terms, that if I wanted my swing and shoulder turn to be longer, I needed to increase my flexibility. It was that simple.

The most impressive thing about this meeting was that, for the first time, someone was able to answer all of the questions that I had about my golf swing. Roger explained in detail the relationship of the body and the golf swing. It was an eye-opener.

If my lack of flexibility was the bad news, there was also good news. Roger was adamant in his belief that I could regain a tremendous amount of flexibility and radically improve my golf swing if I followed his program diligently. Shortly thereafter, I flew him down to Bay Hill in Orlando, where we started my training in earnest.

I strongly recommend that you follow Roger's instructions in this book, as I am confident that you will experience the amazing benefits that his wonderful program has given to me and thousands of others.

Although Roger has designed this program for golf, there is no doubt that it will also carry over into your life away from the golf course. I only wish I had started it 20 years ago.

I am honored to help Roger promote this powerful message. What we are trying to do is make the greatest game on Earth even more enjoyable for everyone who plays it.

—*Arnold Palmer*

PROLOGUE: THE 400-YEAR-OLD MYSTERY

FOR MORE THAN 400 YEARS, the game of golf has been one of the most mysterious and fascinating pursuits ever invented by mankind. From Scottish sheepherders to modern-day athletes, from laborers to executives, from heads of state to the common man, people are fascinated by golf. It seems to seize the imagination and scramble the mind of every person who plays it, or has ever played it. Yet after all these decades, the debate on what is the "right way" or the "best method" to swing a golf club still exists. In fact, there is more technology and more golf instruction "tips" and lessons than ever before! Thousands of books and magazine articles have been written on the subject. Endless videos have been produced. Many instructors want to provide the secret for improving our golf games. Regardless, there is no conclusive proof that one way is better than another way. There is no compelling evidence that a particular way is absolutely the right way.

Some teachers have told us to turn our hips, while others have told us to quiet them. Some have told us to cup our wrists; others have told us to keep them flat. They have told us to swing upright; they have told us to get our swing on plane. They have told us to keep our elbow in tight; they have told us to let it fly. They have told us this, and they have told us that. But what they seldom tell us is this: Despite the remarkable advancements in golf technology, golf instruction, and golf course conditioning, handicaps have scarcely come down over the past 30 years. In other words, the overwhelming majority of golfers haven't improved.

THERE'S NO ONE RIGHT WAY TO SWING A GOLF CLUB

The truth is obvious: If we take a look at golf's all-time greatest players, it is clear there is no absolute correct way to swing a golf club *(Figs. P.1–P.3).* There have been great players who played with strong grips, weak grips, neutral grips, crisscross grips, long thumb, short thumb, overlap, interlock, and 10-finger, and even a few gifted players who played with cross-hand grips. There have been players who set their wrists early, players who took the club back in one piece, and players who dragged it back. There have been inside takeaways, straight-back takeaways, and outside loopy takeaways. There have been upright planes, neutral planes, and flat planes. There have been cupped wrists, flat wrists, and convex wrists. Since there have been great players who played with each one of these characteristics, who's to say which way is the right way?

THE GREATEST SECRET NEVER TOLD

Looking at all the swing mechanics and tips that golf instructors are passing along to their students, people have naturally assumed that all they have to do is incorporate that particular tip, keep repeating it, and then they're going to be the golfer they've always dreamed of being. The reality is, however, that not all golfers can do it. Some can, but many can't. If your body is not flexible enough to accommodate a certain movement, you probably will introduce a compensating swing mistake in your attempt to make that movement.

Most instructors unschooled in flexibility invariably tell their students to keep working

Fig. P.1 Laid off

Fig. P.2 Down the line

Fig. P.3 Across the line

on it. It should be clear that in many cases this is a myth. In fact, in many if not most cases, when a golfer keeps on "grooving" a swing tip that they physically can't do, they're actually perfecting their faults. If everybody could do it, then everybody would be improving—and most people don't improve. The teachers often blame it on lack of practice or poor practice habits, but I'm saying there's another reason.

LACK OF FLEXIBILITY: THE BIGGEST PROBLEM IN GOLF

Electromyographic research has proven that PGA Tour players possess 50 to 100 percent more flexibility in their upper trunks than average golfers. Furthermore, they possess about a two-thirds faster pelvic rotation through the shot than the average golfer. There is no doubt in my mind that lack of flexibility is the number one problem in golf. Most golfers, even some with a high degree of skill, are plagued by their inability to move their bodies in an effective and efficient manner. As a result, they are tormented by their failure to achieve prescribed positions in the golf swing.

The reason for this is no mystery. Humans today have lifestyles that are largely sedentary. We sit at our jobs, sit in our cars, and sit at home in front of our televisions. As a result, our bodies become anatomically dysfunctional, and we take these same dysfunctional bodies to the golf course. And then we bogey our brains out. Our sedentary/sitting-down lifestyle has weakened some muscles, tightened others, and greatly affected the capacity of many individuals to make a proper golf swing. After all, the golf swing is a complex athletic move. It is gymnastic in its demands on the human body. Most golfers simply do not possess the flexibility to get into the positions that their instructors want. In many cases, trying to get their dysfunctional bodies into functional positions only makes them worse!

THE FUTURE OF GOLF INSTRUCTION

Many golf teachers do not recognize the fragile relationship between the human body and the golf swing. If students repeatedly are asked to do things they cannot do, they become frustrated. Often they get angry—with themselves, with their teachers, or with the game of golf itself. No wonder golf has flatlined, with the number of new golfers not matching the number of golfers leaving the game. This frustration is exactly what golf does not need. Golf is supposed to be relaxing. It is supposed to be engrossing. It is supposed to be fun. There is no room for anger.

Frankly, I feel that golf has become way too complicated! Despite the fact that I've been in the golf world for more than 50 years, I was recently taken aback at a visit to the PGA Merchandise Show in Orlando. What amazed me was how technical the game has gotten, especially in golf instruction. Whether it was in the incredible new research in 3-D motion sensors, ongoing teaching philosophies, training aids, smartphones with video-training systems, and so forth, I left there thinking that the golf instruction industry was looking at golfers as if they were robots rather than human beings who have feelings, nerves, emotions, muscle imbalances, and poor posture. Although golf is probably the hardest sport on the planet, in reality it's not *that* complicated. I've been very blessed to have worked with many of the greatest golfers that have ever lived, and believe me when I say that most of them didn't really know that much about the golf swing—as compared to what's going on now. True, most of the players I'm referring to grew up in an era that didn't have all this technology; they mainly played by feel and by developing their own kinesthetic awareness. And feel, along with balance, rhythm, and timing are things that I think have gotten lost in today's technical golf world.

I believe there is a new dawn rising in the golf instruction world. I believe that the instructors of the future will recognize how a person's body affects the ability to make a golf swing. The instructors of the future will be aware of their students' posture types, their ranges of motion, their strength and athleticism. Golf instructors of the LPGA and PGA will know as much about hip flexors as they do about high fades. They will teach golf, of course, but they will also be experts in flexibility exercises and fitness. They will be aware of their students' limitations before they prescribe golf swing mechanics, and they will know what their students can and cannot do.

Think about it. Think how diligently you tried to make that shoulder turn or some other move. There might have been a voice inside you that said, "This is hard. This doesn't feel good. Can this possibly be right?" If so, then perhaps you should have paid attention to that voice. The answer to this dilemma does not lie only in swing instruction. It also lies in regular flexibility training, followed by some strength and cardiovascular training. What happens to golfers who do not possess the necessary flexibility to perform a fundamental golf swing? The answer is simple: Their bodies make some kind of compensation in an attempt to rectify this lack of flexibility.

If you can't turn your shoulders properly on the backswing, your body will find a way to compensate by moving other body parts. You might rise up, your rear leg may straighten, or your lower body may slide and lose its stability. You might feel as if you are doing it right, but video analysis and especially 3-D motion-capture systems *(Fig. P.4)* always expose the truth. Com-

Fig P.4 3-D motion-capture systems are revealing many truths about what the body is doing during the golf swing motion.

pensations in the golf swing invariably lead to a loss of stability at some point during the swing. Lose your stability and your center of balance and you have lost the war to the golf demons.

Flexibility is the answer. Flexibility will lead to a sound, repeatable golf swing. This book is all about incorporating sound golf instruction principles with flexibility training exercises. The intent is to make your body more flexible so that your golf swing will be more flexible.

THE GOOD NEWS

The good news is that everybody, no matter their age, can improve the range of motion in their bodies by stretching the right muscles in the right way. When we improve the range of motion in our bodies, we automatically improve the range of motion in our swings—pure and simple.

I incorporated these principles into my own life more than 20 years ago, and they have literally transformed my body and my golf swing.

Now, at age 59, I am more flexible than I ever was in my teens, twenties, or thirties. Believe me when I say this: You don't have to lose flexibility as you get older. In fact, you can gain a considerable amount of flexibility if you do the right stretches the right way.

During the past 2 decades, I have exposed tens of thousands of people to these principles and have received great joy from watching them reconstruct their bodies and their golf swings. They have rediscovered a fountain of youth, if you will. It is my goal to redirect the thinking of the legions of golfers who play this wonderful game and help them realize the potential and joy that dwells within them.

You can make a bigger shoulder turn, you can learn to control your body, and you can increase your flexibility!

In addition, you can realize the greatest gift that any golfer can ever receive—a freer and more powerful golf swing. I know you can do this because I see people improve every day at my golf instruction schools.

CHAPTER 1

MY STORY

"YOU MUST HAVE ONE HECK OF A SORE LEFT ANKLE WHEN YOU HIT A LOT OF GOLF BALLS." Those words were uttered to me in 1985 by a physical therapist named Ric McDonald, who at the time was the head trainer for the San Diego Chargers football team. Although I didn't know it then, that one sentence would change the course of my life and would actually start me out on a new career.

That sentence became so important to me that it is etched in my memory. Ric said it just as I was reaching for the doorknob to leave his office. We had just concluded a business meeting that had nothing to do with physical therapy or golf. Flabbergasted, I turned to him and asked, "How did you know that?"

"Look at your posture," he said. My posture at the time was horrible. I had severe rotation in my hips, and my right shoulder was rounded and pulled down and forward (like with many golfers). He explained the body's natural and correct posture, and he showed me how severely out of balance I was. From there, Ric described my golf swing tendencies and pinpointed precisely how my poor posture was contributing to my swing faults. He explained in detail how my tight right hip and impinged right shoulder were inhibiting my ability to turn my right side on my backswing, how the lack of extension in my right wrist (due to a prosthetic) was forcing the club open, and how my weaker left hip didn't have the ability to stabilize properly as I shifted my weight onto it in the downswing, thus forcing me to spin out, which in turn forced my left foot to roll to the outside, causing me pain. (I remember thinking, "So that's why I've had so many left ankle problems!")

I was *shocked*. He had never seen me before, let alone seen me swing a golf club. Yet his diagnosis was absolutely right on. It was like he had a supernatural gift. I was amazed. It was the start of a grand awakening. For the first time, I realized I might be able to end a lifetime of confusion about the golf swing. I might be able to find answers to questions that had been plaguing me since I was a kid.

THE BEGINNING

My life in golf started back in Santa Barbara, California, where I grew up. At about age 7, I began following my father, Elmer Fredericks, around the golf course. He was a fine player with a beautiful swing and could hit the ball a mile. I eventually got my first set of clubs—Bobby Jones Juniors. There were two woods, four irons, and a putter. Like most kids starting out, I'd take a wide stance and give it a hockey slap shot type of motion down the fairway.

When I was 9, my father got me a complete set of First Flight clubs. I couldn't wait for them to arrive. My anticipation was off the charts. They were too long for me, but my dad said they would be fine and that soon enough I'd grow into them. I immediately went out to play with them at La Cumbre Country Club, where my parents were members, and I couldn't have hit the ball any worse if I had tried. The new clubs felt terrible. I was demoralized. My dad had left work early and joined me in the middle of the fourth fairway to see how I was doing with the new clubs. What he found was a very disconsolate son.

He told me to hit a few balls so he could figure out why I was hitting bad shots. He watched for a few minutes, and then he confidently said, "I've got it! I know exactly what is happening. Because the clubs are longer, you're going to need to take it back longer so you can create more leverage." He told me to take the club back low and slow, and swing it back as far as possible—and wait for it at the top. His advice produced a much longer, rhythmic swing. Up until then, I had a very short backswing that had worked just fine with my old set, but it wasn't well suited for these longer clubs.

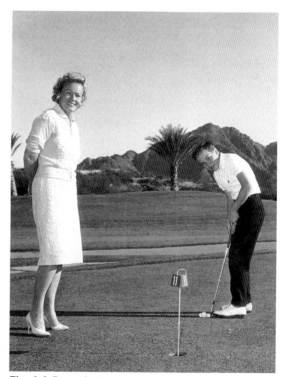

Fig. 1.1 Roger in the early days

THE MAGIC MOMENT

This actually was my first lesson, and it changed my relationship with golf. It was unbelievable. Every shot I hit was high and long. From that moment, I became compulsive—amazed that by simply making one little change in my swing I could make such a profound difference! I had discovered the magic that is legendary in golf. That particular day was the beginning of my search for the secrets of the golf swing.

Most golfers, I have come to realize, are looking for this magic in their games. Nearly all golfers spend their lives searching for some swing secrets, or that one little thing that will make a difference. Everybody goes through this, from Joe Hacker to golf's greatest players. I see this all the time in my golf schools, and it never fails to remind me of that day when I first found the magic in the company of my father. I remember it vividly: the flight of the ball, the consistency of my shots, and the absolute joy of discovering that one little thing that made such a dramatic difference.

There is purity and innocence in this joy, and it is something I see frequently in my students. We can be incredibly successful as adults and yet, at the same time, we can retain that childlike quality of excitement and zeal about golf.

The game of golf offers a lifetime of discoveries—new swing tips that lead to the overwhelming feeling that we've finally got *it* and *it* won't go away. Even when *it* disappears, as *it* inevitably does, we can get *it* back. Golf, after all, is a quest that never ends. Looking back now, I realize that magic moment with my father was the start of my golf instructional

odyssey. It didn't take me long to become one of the greatest golf swing psycho junkies who ever lived. There wasn't a round of golf that I played when I wasn't trying something new or different, and this pattern went on for decades.

ADDICTED TO GOLF LESSONS

As a junior golfer, I took lessons from several renowned teachers, but ultimately I still played by feel. I received a partial golf scholarship to Arizona State University, which had (and still has) one of the top college golf programs in the country.

In 1972, after college, I turned professional and worked hard on my game in preparation for the PGA qualifying school in the fall. In June of that year, I suffered a very serious wrist injury, which eventually required two major surgeries. In the first surgery, doctors did a bone graft, taking bone out of my hip and transplanting it into my wrist. That surgery failed and my wrist got worse. In the next surgery, a year or so later, they literally cut one of my metacarpal bones in half and inserted a prosthetic (which is still there today). The recovery process took more than a year and a half, and I was in a cast much of that time. When I was finally able to resume playing, I noticed a tremendous difference in the way I hit the ball. What I discovered was that my old reliable right-to-left draw, the shot I had hit all my life, was completely gone. It was replaced by a weak push-fade that really didn't go anywhere. My accuracy was gone, too, along with my confidence.

This confused me terribly. To get back on

the right track, I sought golf instruction from anyone and everyone. I took lessons from a legion of teachers. You name them, I probably went to them. If I didn't see them, I read their books or watched their videos, or I picked the brains of people who had seen them. I tried everything imaginable. Even more confusing was that many of these teachers had opposing theories about the golf swing. These theories often conflicted with each other so much that I became entirely confused. When I say I took lessons from them, I don't mean an occasional lesson here or there. I mean I worked at it. I'd sometimes hit 500 balls a day trying to groove what they were teaching me.

I also trained with Chinese martial arts teachers to learn and adapt energy transfer and power concepts to the golf swing. More than once, I persuaded a Chinese kung fu master to try to figure out the golf swing. Each one was as fascinated and confused as I was.

Claude Harmon and Paul Runyan were two of the great instructors whom I saw for several years. Although both were incredibly knowledgeable, their teaching concepts were diametrically opposed. For example, Claude wanted me to play with a weak left-hand grip; Paul wanted a strong left-hand position. Claude advocated a wide stance; Paul liked a narrow stance. Claude told me to keep my hands high at address; Paul wanted them low. Claude wanted me to set my wrists early; Paul wanted me to drag the club back. You get the picture? And that was just to address and start the swing. When it came to the full swing, I was unable to simplify things. Every teacher had a different theory.

I wouldn't be surprised if I drove many of these teachers to their psychiatrists' couches

because of the countless questions I asked. While I listened and tried to learn each system, I couldn't help but notice that a high percentage of great players had unorthodox swings. Furthermore, their swings were so distinctive that seldom did you ever see any two people swing the same way. Just look at the swings of Arnold Palmer, Lee Trevino, Chi Chi Rodriguez, Doug Sanders, Miller Barber, Jim Furyk, and others, and you'll see what I mean.

There were dozens of great players whose golf swings weren't even close to each other. I'd watch very successful players with short swings and long swings, strong grips and weak grips, early wrist sets and one-piece takeaways, cupped wrists and flat wrists, upright swings and flat swings. I would often go to my teachers and say something like, "You know, I was watching Lee Trevino and Gene Littler play the other day, and their swings are completely different. They don't do what you're telling me to do."

Most teachers would tell me those players were exceptions. That made sense at the time. Yet, it never occurred to me that maybe *I* was an exception. In fact, maybe we're all exceptions and are all "uniquely unique."

CLUELESS ABOUT THE GOLF SWING

This instructional journey lasted for nearly 12 years, and my golf game went from PGA Tour material to an 8-handicap. The odds were 50-50 if I would break 80 on any given day. I can honestly say that, after all the different methods and all the different teachers, nobody made me a better golfer. Nobody gave me the "secret" or made me feel confident in my skills. In fact, I got so confused that I was literally lost in a maze from which there was no escape. I barely knew which end of the club to hold. I thought of quitting the game all the time, but I couldn't. I was a psychological mess.

I didn't realize at the time that all my experiences—as a player and especially as a student of all these great teachers—would eventually help me become a better instructor. Everything I went through—all the joy and frustration—would motivate me to understand the complexities of the golf swing. I feel strongly that to be a good teacher, one has to experience much of this to be able to comprehend what is happening inside the minds and bodies of one's students. Golf is a perplexing mental game, and an excellent instructor has to be a psychologist and a motivator, as well as a master of the golf swing.

DOCTORS AND FAITH HEALERS

To complicate the situation, my body began to deteriorate as I struggled with my golf game. My left knee was painful all the time. This required two knee surgeries to go along with my two wrist surgeries. Occasionally, I suffered from shooting sciatica that would sear down my hip and legs. I didn't know what I was going to do with my life.

The story of my body parallels the story of my golf swing. That is, I went to everybody to fix my knee pain. You name them, I've been to them—orthopedic surgeons, physical therapists, Rolfists, chiropractors, deep-tissue mas-

sage therapists, acupuncturists, acupressurists, martial artists, even a Filipino faith healer (who actually helped by explaining to me that my knee problem was a symptom of my misaligned hips). And, just like with my golf swing, nobody or any of their treatments provided a definitive answer. In fact, with each passing year, my knee got worse and worse until my left patella (kneecap) would literally slide off of its track.

Despite all this, I never gave up the dream of playing on the PGA Tour. I worked very hard on my game with the intent of someday, somehow, making it to the Tour. I never gave up that dream—until I played a round of golf one day with Craig Stadler.

THE CRAIG STADLER DECISION

I was invited to play with Craig Stadler at La Jolla Country Club near San Diego. Craig arrived at the course about 1 minute before our tee time and didn't hit one warmup shot. He went straight from the parking lot to the first tee. Despite missing two 20-inch putts, he shot the easiest 65 that I've ever seen. And he didn't seem elated at all. In fact, he seemed like he didn't even care. If that had been me, I would've been celebrating for weeks. Even the good rounds that I had shot seemed like hard work. Never had I shot a round with the ease that he had—and I had been practicing my game for years. Right then I experienced a moment of clarity. I asked myself, "What in the world am I trying to do?" And right then I gave up my dream of playing on the PGA Tour. That decision turned out to be a good thing because fate had something else in mind.

THE MEN WHO CHANGED THE DIRECTION OF MY LIFE

By the time I met Ric McDonald, he had been the head trainer of the San Diego Chargers for 19 years. His reputation in the field of physical therapy was legendary. He had recently joined forces with a unique anatomical functionalist named Pete Egoscue (who eventually became Jack Nicklaus's trainer and opened the internationally renowned Egoscue clinics).

Ric and Pete teamed up to start a physical therapy clinic called T.H.E. (Therapy, Health, and Education) Clinic, in Del Mar, California, and I was lucky enough to become associated with them. As Ric explained to me why all the golf lessons hadn't worked on my swing, he also explained why all the therapy hadn't worked on my knee. The cause of both problems lay in my poor posture, which in turn was related to the muscle imbalances in my body. These muscle imbalances were also the cause of the problems in my golf swing mechanics. Ric explained to me precisely how "your body is your golf swing," and that until I straightened out my posture, I would continue to have problems, and that even future surgeries wouldn't help.

As he was speaking, I was literally in awe and somewhat in a state of shock. I had never even thought about the possibility that my body was the cause of the flaws in my golf swing. I had never associated one with the other.

I, like so many people, had always subscribed to the mistaken belief that by just working on swing mechanics I was going to improve my golf swing. Just working on golf swing mechanics, however, isn't necessarily going to grow you a new hamstring or increase the length of your hip flexors! This is the very myth that I've been trying to dispel for more than 25 years now. It is the foundation of my entire message today. I had never even thought of that concept before! I distinctly remember telling myself at the time that this guy knew more about the truth of the golf swing than all of the instructors I had seen put together—and this coming from a 14-handicap no less! I was finally learning the truth about the golf swing.

Finally, I asked him, "Can you fix my knee?" He looked me right in the eye and said, "Oh, yeah, that's a piece of cake. And by the way, your knee isn't your problem; it's your hips. Your knees don't track directly underneath your hips because of the dominance of your right hip, which has caused your pelvis to rotate to the left. As long as your hips are out of alignment, your knee will never get better." He went on to tell me that if I followed his advice, I'd not only be pain-free in a short amount of time, but I'd be running and jumping with no pain. Again I was astounded, because every health practitioner had told me that running was bad for my knees.

Ric told me that, for me, this wasn't true. He said that once he loosened the muscles of my legs and hips and began a proper flexibility and posture-restoration program, my pelvis would be able to float and my knees would track directly underneath, where they were designed to be. He went on to explain that when my knees were once again tracking directly underneath my hips, I could run to my heart's content.

FIXING MY KNEES

The next week we got together, and Ric began to put me through a type of therapy that I'd never seen before. He instructed me to do a gravity-relaxation exercise (the supine groin stretch, S54, page 193) along with some unusual poses and stretches. Within 45 minutes, I could feel the pain leaving my knee. This was magic in itself, and I carefully followed his instructions for the next several months.

Just like he said, in a short amount of time I had no pain. I became dedicated to increasing my flexibility and getting my body back in postural alignment. I started feeling lighter, taller, and more confident. And guess what? As my body began to improve, my golf game began to improve. Within a year and a half after embarking on this program, I set one course record in San Diego and tied another! Let's see here, I used to be young and in good shape and played excellent golf. Then I got way out of shape and played poor golf. Then I got back into good shape again and played excellent golf! Hmmm. Even a fool could see this was no coincidence!

At once, I began to learn this philosophy as fast as I could. I couldn't get enough. While I was learning about the body—and specifically my body—I began to learn other things as well, including the following:

- Why so many people struggle with their golf games because they don't understand their bodies.

- How the muscles influence the golf swing.

- Why handicaps have scarcely (if at all) come down in 30 years despite the remarkable advances in golf club technology, teaching, and course conditioning.

- How the golf swing is definitely an athletic movement that requires ample flexibility and strength in the key muscle groups.

THE INFLUENCE OF JACK NICKLAUS

My learning process became more intense after Ric and Pete created their T.H.E. Clinic. In the first few months, Jack Nicklaus came to visit Pete to be treated for his ailing back. When Pete and Jack had completed their session, Jack asked Pete what he could do about his flying right elbow, which is still one of the most famous moves in the history of golf.

Pete explained that Jack's flying right elbow was merely a symptom of his tight rhomboid muscles, which inhibited his shoulder blades and forced his right elbow to flare out. I watched in wonder as Jack's eyes opened wide. He too became enlightened upon discovering that his swing mechanics were a direct result of his anatomical function. For the first time, he understood why so many of the external swing remedies hadn't worked for him, either. Jack relayed to us how he had tried virtually everything to keep his elbow closer to his side to remain more connected through his backswing, including drills using a head cover under his armpit and straps around his arms.

I watched in amazement as the greatest player of all time told us his story about his struggle to fix this element of his swing. Finally, Jack said something to the effect of, "You know, Pete, this is powerful stuff. I want to help you get the message out there about the importance of anatomical function in the golf swing."

Right then I knew what I wanted to do with my life and career: I wanted to help get this powerful message out to the golf world—that the golf swing is an athletic movement requiring flexibility and strength in the key muscle groups, that people should address the sport from an anatomical perspective, and that simply practicing golf swing mechanics is usually not enough.

SPREADING THE MESSAGE

Eventually, I opened my own golf school, and I started spreading the message that the average person doesn't possess enough flexibility to perform a fundamental golf swing. I've been doing this now for more than 25 years, and the world finally seems attentive. Several years after I began preaching golf fitness, Tiger Woods came along and took it to a level never seen before. Years after that, Wally Uihlein, the CEO of Acushnet Company, recruited Dr. Greg Rose and Dave Phillips and created the Titleist Performance Institute. Today, it isn't just a few people who are listening. Serious golfers everywhere seem to understand that the modern lifestyle hinders their golf swings. They are savvy enough to know they need help. I hear people talk all the time about the modern golf swing. I find it so interesting that the modern golf swing is the direct opposite of the modern lifestyle. The modern swing is a very athletic move that requires plenty of flexibility; yet the modern lifestyle reduces our flexibility and tightens our bodies. Since joining forces with Ric McDonald and Pete Egoscue, my entire philosophy has been based on coordinating the development of the body with the mechanics of the golf swing. There is no doubt in my mind that this is the 21st-century approach to golf, and I am a very lucky person to be part of this movement. Today, there is no doubt, the golf fitness movement is alive and well. And it is here to stay.

POSTURE AND BALANCE: WE ARE ALL CREATED EQUAL

THE FOUNDATION OF YOUR BODY (AND YOUR GOLF SWING)

People are different. We come in varied shapes, sizes, colors, heights, and weights. In other words, we are all "uniquely unique." It is this uniqueness that makes each and every one of us special, and it is this uniqueness that makes life so interesting. Whether hobbies, interests, politics, or even our golf swings, the differences among people make our world go round. Despite our infinitely varied traits, however, there is one aspect in which all of us are created equal: The musculoskeletal design of the human body is the same for everybody. With the exception of a small number of people who are born with deformities, our bodies are designed with the same blueprint. We are born with this design, and providing that we use and work our bodies properly, it will not change. If we guard and protect this design, we will function properly and efficiently in everything that we do.

HUNTERS AND GATHERERS

Our bodies were designed by the Creator to be hunters and gatherers. Each muscle and fiber of our being was designed to be in motion from sunrise to sunset, constantly moving. Combined with proper walking, bending, reaching, dragging, and so forth, we were designed for activities such as reaping crops, planting seeds, picking fruit, walking up hills, and straddling creeks. In other words, we were designed to be in motion.

When our ancestors lived this way in the wild, their constant motion resulted in strong and stable feet; powerful and pliable legs; hips that efficiently synchronized the lower and upper bodies; strong arms, chest, and shoul-

Fig. 2.1 We are all designed to be in motion.

ders; and a head that sat squarely on top of the shoulders. Their lifestyle of hunting and gathering contributed to their overall condition, which was one of strength, flexibility, balance, and perfect posture.

MODERN CIVILIZATION AND THE DECLINE OF THE HUMAN BODY

Around the start of the 20th century, with the onset of the Industrial Age, the lifestyle and environment of our species took a radical turn. Rather than hunt and gather, or walk and roam like our ancestors did in the wild *(Fig. 2.1)*, the vast majority of the population began a lifestyle that is now altering the integrity of our design. We began to move less and sit down more *(Figs. 2.2–2.4)*. As a result, the human body began to evolve out of its natural design and become out of balance. The perfect symmetry and synchronization of the muscles is now being compromised.

When we sit down, the powerful hip flexor muscles are actually being exercised because they're supporting the upper trunk as it tilts forward. As a result, the hip muscles begin to shorten and tighten and tend to pull the pelvis forward. Not only does this increase the forward (or anterior) tilt of the pelvis, but one side of the pelvis usually becomes more dominant than the other (usually the right side).

Think about the process of driving a car. First we sit down in the seat. Then we engage in the repetitive use of our right foot and leg, moving from the accelerator to the brake millions of times over a lifetime. This can dramatically strengthen and tighten the right hip and

Fig. 2.2 Whether we are sitting at our desks . . .

force it out of balance with the left. Coupled with the excessive anterior tilt, the pelvis will also become rotated due to the dominance and overuse of one side of the hip. If that's not bad enough, as we sit down more and more in our daily lives, our shoulders begin to lean forward and become rounded. The result is that the majority of people in our culture are out of nature's design.

Fig. 2.3 . . . in our cars . . .

Fig. 2.4 . . . or on our couches, the sedentary lifestyle plays havoc on our bodies and our golf swings.

THE DESIGN

The proper posture and design of the human body is as follows: From a face-on view *(Fig. 2.5)*, we should see the hip joints over the knees and the knees over the feet, which should point straight ahead. The shoulder joints should stack up on top of the hip joints, and the head should be directly in the middle of the body, right on top of the sternum. From the side view *(Fig. 2.6)*, we should see the ear over the shoulder, the shoulder over the hip, the hip over the knee, and the knee over the ankle. The four joints plus the ear should be in direct vertical alignment with each other. Unfortunately, we don't see many people in perfect alignment these days. What we normally see are the three posture types described on opposite page.

Primarily due to the sedentary/sitting-down lifestyle and the repetitive stress of certain activities, over the past century, the structural design of the human body has been compromised. When the integrity of the design is

Fig. 2.5 Face-on view displaying perfect posture

Fig. 2.6 Side view

Fig. 2.7 Rounded shoulders/ forward head posture

Fig. 2.8 C-curve/under posture

Fig. 2.9 Rotated posture

affected, the entire system is affected. The hip girdle changes its tilt, the spine changes its curve, and the entire body begins to compensate—creating misalignments. For example, for every inch that the head sits forward of the center line, one is adding around 12 pounds of stress to every ligament, tendon, and organ of the body *(Fig. 2.10)*.

12 lbs.   32 lbs.   42 lbs.

1 INCH FORWARD   2 INCHES FORWARD   3 INCHES FORWARD

Fig. 2.10

THE IMPORTANCE OF POSTURE AND YOUR GOLF SWING

Posture Type 1: **Rounded Shoulders/ Forward Head**

This posture type is probably the most common in our culture. When you see this posture, with the hips, shoulders, and head leaning forward, you know that the individual has tight and shortened muscles, primarily in the hips and upper torso. Because gravity is in essence pulling the body forward, the upper-back muscles tighten to keep the torso upright and prevent it from falling down, much like a rider pulling the reins to slow down a horse. Once again, our sitting-down lifestyle, along with bending over so much doing activities, is the cause. From the side view *(Fig. 2.11)*, one only has to notice the position of the ears in relation to the hip joint, and also the angle of the hips, which are tilted forward. Again, the ear, shoulder, hip, knee, and ankle were designed to be in vertical alignment. From the face-on view *(Fig. 2.12)*, you'll normally see everted feet (the old Charlie Chaplain look). Because of the muscle tightness in the hip flexors and the upper torso, the pelvis begins to pull inward.

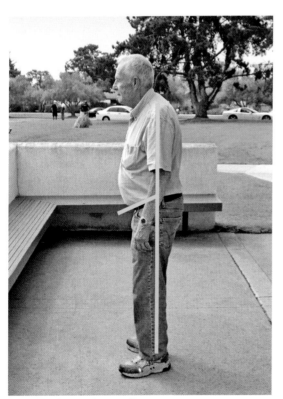

Fig. 2.11 Forward torso tilt

Fig. 2.12 Everted feet due to tight and imbalanced hips

Fig. 2.13 Weight on heels, rounded shoulders due to tight hips and upper torso

Fig. 2.14 Notice how the hip joint stacks directly on top of the ankle, indicating perfect balance.

Fig. 2.15 Flat shoulder plane due to tight chest muscles

Fig. 2.16 Arnold Palmer demonstrating a perfect shoulder plane

The feet in turn tend to flare out in an effort to counterbalance the forces of the hips. Another condition often associated with rounded shoulders/forward head posture is internal and/or external rotation of the femurs, which then put friction on the hip, knee, and ankle joints. This creates a phenomenon called tibial and femoral torsion, which again is symptomatic of imbalances primarily in the hips. When you see everted feet, you know that imbalances exist in the hips—which will then carry over into one's golf swing.

The *best* thing to do for this condition is to begin a program involving proper flexibility and posture-restoration exercises to get "out of flexion" and into a more erect and functional posture.

When a muscle becomes too short or tight, it's simply not going to be able to stretch and elongate. Consequently, people with this posture type will usually have a hard time expanding the chest or achieving a functional hip and shoulder turn. These restrictions often cause swing faults such as staying down into the shot, restricted shoulder turns, chicken wings, and straightening of the legs.

EFFECTS ON THE GOLF SWING This posture type prevents a golfer from staying down into the shot and restricts hip turns or straightens the legs *(Fig. 2.19)*. In addition, the tightness in the shoulders and pectoral muscles (pecs) restricts the upper torso's expansion in both the backswing and the forward swing.

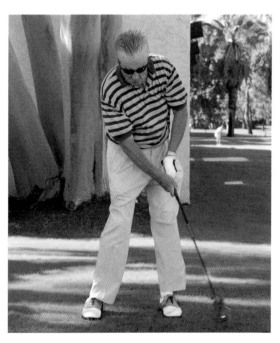

Fig. 2.17 Restricted hip shift due to tight hips

Fig. 2.18 Flexible hips allow the torso to shift on to the front foot

Fig. 2.19 Straightening of the legs due to lower-body tightness

WHAT TO DO

• NARROW THE STANCE A wider stance tends to restrict movement, and since this posture type is indicative of restricted and tight muscles, I recommend a narrow stance. For a drill on narrowing the stance, see D22 on page 117.

• STRENGTHEN THE LEFT-HAND GRIP Because this posture type has restricted muscles, it's advisable to allow the hands to have more play in the swing. Strengthening the left-hand grip (for right-handers) will create more wrist action and help make up for the lack of motion in the torso. For a drill on strengthening the grip, see D24 on page 119.

• STAND TALLER The more a person is bent over (as forward posture types are), the harder it is for the body to rotate and move. Standing taller will help the person move easier and not force

the body into unnecessary compensations. I can't stress this swing tip enough! For a drill on standing taller, see D23 on page 118.

For a functional body and a functional golf swing, we need muscles that elongate or stretch. In my view, a short and tightened muscle doesn't move very well, and a muscle that doesn't move is a weak muscle. Weak and imbalanced muscles inhibit the golf swing motion. The secret to reversing this posture is not necessarily stretching out the chest or strengthening the back, but rather relaxing and stretching the hips and strengthening the glutes.

Posture Type 2: **C-Curve/Under**

This posture type is quite common in the elderly and is defined simply as being *weak* and unstable. As you can see *(Fig. 2.20)*, the hips are tilted upward, indicating that there's simply

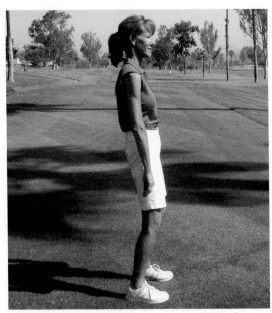

Fig. 2.20 C-curve/under posture due to lack of strength in the lower body

not enough strength and support from the legs (and hips). The powerful hip flexor muscles, which we rely on so heavily in our bodies, simply have gotten too weak to do their job, which is to support the upper torso. In this weak and unstable position, the shoulders tilt forward to counterbalance the under position of the hips. Another characteristic of the C-curve/under posture is the head jutting forward to counterbalance the effects of the center of gravity.

EFFECTS ON THE GOLF SWING Due to the lack of strength and muscle tightness in the lower body, a golfer with this posture type will lack stability, which will usually result in the golfer losing the brace of their stance, that is if they even got into a braced address position to begin with. They will tend to help the club up by lifting it with the upper torso *(Figs. 2.21 and 2.22)* rather than allowing the trunk to shift the weight in balance and swing the arms freely. Consequently, you'll see a swing where the arms run amok and flail. It's one thing to be an arms type of player, but you want the entire body working in unison (the legs, hips, torso, shoulders, and arms).

As for the type of shots, don't expect to see any solid shots or power here. The power is generated by the coiling of the upper trunk against the resistance and bracing of the lower body,

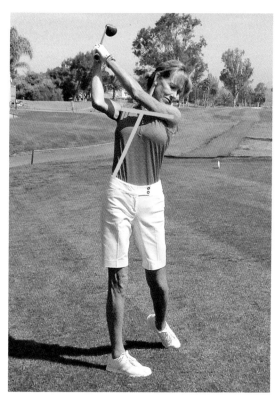

Fig. 2.21 Standing up and coming out of the spine angle due to a lack of lower-body stability

Fig. 2.22 A great example of lower-body stability allowing a consistent spine angle

and then uncoiling this power through the arms and hands. Using just the hands and arms isn't enough! Tops, skulls, scuffs, and shanks are normally the outcome of this posture type.

WHAT TO DO

• **STRENGTHEN THE GRIP** Because of the lack of strength in the torso, you should strengthen the left-hand grip (if you are a right-hander) to create more power out of the wrists. For a drill on strengthening the grip, see D24 on page 119.

• **WIDEN THE STANCE** Although I generally don't prefer wide stances, we've got to get some lower-body stability into the C-curve posture's golf swing. Widening the stance will create much needed stability in the foundation. This will also help curb the "lifting" that is almost sure to occur. For a drill on widening the stance, see D25 on page 120.

• **SET, TURN, AND PLACE DRILL** This drill will help develop a good feel of blending the wrists, arms, and turn into the swing, and it should help (along with the solid stance) eliminate the lifting of the torso. For the set, turn, and place drill, see D7 on page 101.

• **SHIFT MORE LATERALLY** The golfer with this posture type will have a hard time maximizing their lower body and shifting onto the front foot. Swinging a power fan or hitting into an Impact Bag are good ways to develop the solid feel of moving into the ball. For drills on shifting laterally, see D17 on page 112 and D18 on page 113.

• **EXERCISE** This person needs to move those legs! Get walking a lot! Walking up stairs forward and backward will strengthen the body tremendously!

Posture Type 3: **Rotated**

I'm not sure if I've ever met a person who didn't have some degree of rotation in the torso—especially in the hips and shoulders. This is particularly evident in athletes who overuse one side of their bodies (tennis players, baseball pitchers, golfers, and so forth). It's pretty easy to understand why, since the overwhelming majority of people are dominant on one side, usually the right side simply because we live in a right-side-dominant world. This condition is especially prevalent in senior golfers. In their case, their rotation is visible by looking at the right shoulder, where you'll usually see a crease in the upper right pec, near the armpit. Another giveaway is looking at their hands from a face-on view. A person who is rotated will nearly always have one hand hanging lower than the other *(Fig. 2.23)*. Although the shoulders are usually most evident, the hips are really the genesis of the problem. By overusing our right sides, including the constant exercising of our right leg and foot while driving, or by doing a semi–lunge squat in our backswings, the hips become overused and, consequently, one side becomes tighter and stronger than the other and begins to overpower the weaker, dysfunctional side. This can create many imbalances, such as one shoulder forward and/or lower than the other, in the hip position. When one side of the pelvis becomes too strong and dominant, the entire body is shifted out of position *(Fig. 2.24)*.

EFFECTS ON THE GOLF SWING The most notable effect on the golf swing with the rotated posture type is that, because these golfers are rotated to the left, they will kinesthetically line up to the right in an attempt to

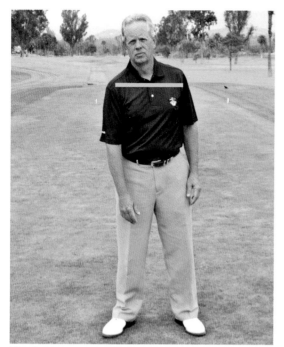

Fig. 2.23 Notice how the dominant right hip has lowered the right shoulder.

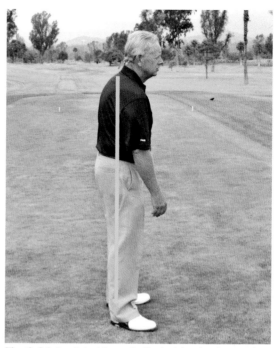

Fig. 2.24 A rotated torso indicated by dominance in the right hip and shoulder

square up their bodies. Not only do they then have to come over the top to hit the ball at the target, but they will normally spin out on the downswing because of the dominance of the right side over the left *(Fig. 2.25)*. The forward-hanging right shoulder also makes it difficult to turn the right side back on the backswing, due to the tightness of the hip and shoulder. Not only does this restrict shoulder turns, but it is often responsible for the dreaded chicken wing, where we see the arms actually collapse. Although the chicken wing looks like an arm problem, the source of the problem is normally found in the lats and shoulders.

LINE UP TO THE RIGHT First off, since this golfer is already rotated left, he will usually

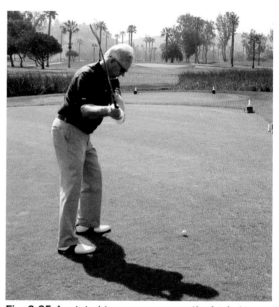

Fig. 2.25 A rotated torso encourages the body to spin out and come over the top.

(and subconsciously) aim to the right, which is a kinesthetic response to squaring himself up. Having lined up to the right, the golfer will now subconsciously know the target is back to the left, and will then tend to come over the top in a subconscious effort to hit the ball toward the target.

OVER THE TOP Because the hips and shoulders are rotated to the left to begin with, the golfer starts out in somewhat of an over-the-top position before she even begins to swing. Lining up to the right and an outside-to-in swing path is imminent.

SPINNING OUT Because of the dominance of the right hip, the weaker left hip and side will usually not want to accept and support the weight being transferred over to them. Instead of the left hip moving somewhat laterally over to the left side before it rotates, it will tend to abbreviate the shift and spin out too early. When the braking action of the body is halted, the club will tend to slow down, creating a hand flip and/or chicken wing through the shot.

This will create a tendency to cut across the ball, with the ball starting out to the left of the target and usually slicing back. "Heeling" the shots is often common with spinning out.

WHAT TO DO

• DRAW YOUR RIGHT FOOT BACK Make sure your alignment is sound, then draw the right foot back (for a right-handed golfer), in a closed position. Drawing the right foot back will certainly help square up the hips and create a more blended turn of the hips and shoulders on the takeaway.

• SQUARE UP YOUR LEFT FOOT Having your left foot slightly flared out is not a bad thing. However, with a rotated (to the left) posture, you're actually enhancing and enabling the left hip to spin out even more. Keeping the left foot relatively square will make it a lot easier to get your left hip over onto your left side—thus encouraging a proper hip shift.

• KEEP YOUR RIGHT SHOULDER BACK AND SWING DOWN FROM THE INSIDE TO THE OUTSIDE A rotated posture with the right shoulder lower and forward tends to force the club shaft out over the top, which in turn forces the left hip to spin out. Keeping the right shoulder back for as long as possible on the downswing forces the left hip to bump laterally over to the left, which ensures the shaft to drop down to the inside.

A DYSFUNCTIONAL BODY INCREASES THE RISK OF INJURY

In all three of these dysfunctional postures, there is one common denominator: The hips have shifted out of position. Once this happens, the entire structure of the body is thrown off. Nearly all injuries—back, knees, hips, shoulders, and feet—occur when the hips have changed position.

Think about it. What's attached to the pelvis? The spine. When the hip shifts, there's going to be friction and pulling with the deep muscles along the spine, leading to back pain, not to mention friction placed on other joints throughout the body.

At the same time, when the hip changes

position, the position of the knee changes, creating stress on the knee (usually in the medial/inside of the knee, leading to knee pain). When the hip position is altered, the head of the femur, which rests in a cavity of the pelvis called the acetabulum, is suddenly rotated. It begins to grind out the synovial fluid and cartilage in the joint. This creates a bone-on-bone scenario. Hello, hip replacement.

For these reasons, we strive to get the body back in its natural four-socket position, with the shoulders, hips, knees, and ankles all lined up. To get there, the pelvis must be restored to its proper position.

PROPER POSTURE COMES FIRST

It all starts with posture—everybody should strive to attain proper posture. It is more than just standing tall and looking better. One definition of posture is a "state of mind." Posture can provide a sense of confidence and well-being. Everything I do is designed to direct people into a better posture. The better their posture in everyday life, the better their posture in their golf swing, and the better they are going to play. It is all related. A balanced, flexible body is the foundation of a fundamental golf swing.

How do we achieve proper posture? By balancing the musculoskeletal system through flexibility and reciprocal-strength programs.

THE FUNDAMENTALS OF THE GOLF SWING

FOR YEARS, I searched for the answer to the golf swing. I was on a quest and sought out countless teaching pros. In the end, I was struck with the simplicity of what I had learned: Throughout golf history, there have been legions of great players that had unorthodox swings. Whenever I would question an instructor, asking why a particular professional didn't swing as the teacher had recommended, the response would usually be something like, "Well, son, they're exceptions. Don't worry about them." Or, "Sure, they swing differently, but they all have good fundamentals." My next question would be, "What are good fundamentals?" Or, "What exactly are the fundamentals?"

As we all know, there are many different theories about the "true" fundamentals of the golf swing. For most of golf's history, the common assessment of these fundamentals has been reasonably clear: Take a good grip, keep your head still, don't look up, keep your left arm straight, return to the address position at impact, and a few others. However, we have learned over the years that the best golfers grip the club in different ways. We have learned that most of them do move their heads, that they do look up (remember, there's a big difference between looking up and coming up), and that the majority of them don't keep the left arm rigid or ramrod straight throughout the swing.

We have learned that none of them return to the address position at impact because both their hips and shoulders are clearly open at ball strike. After years and years, it finally dawned on me that maybe all of us are exceptions to some degree. After all, we are all uniquely unique.

Without question, flexibility should be considered golf's foremost fundamental. Without proper range of motion, golfers have to overcome too many obstacles and make too many compensations throughout their swings. In the world according to Roger, flexibility and range of motion are at the base of a consistent golf swing.

But what about the actual swing? What are the fundamentals?

MY THREE GOLF DISCOVERIES

Once I was exposed to high-speed video cameras, I began to understand the golf swing with much more clarity. Right away I made three discoveries.

1. It is impossible to give an accurate lesson with the naked eye.
2. There is no one "right way" to swing a golf club.
3. What people think and feel they are doing is seldom what they are actually doing.

As teaching pro Butch Harmon frequently says, "The feel is seldom real." All my life, I have been fascinated by great golf and great golfers. I have tried to be a keen observer of what these players are doing. The key, though, was watching hundreds (if not thousands) of hours of videotape. Pros around San Diego had amassed huge amounts of videotape of top players, and finally it was possible to dispel many of the old myths about the golf swing.

My experience has taught me, and these vid-

eotapes confirmed, that there are really only three true fundamentals, all of which apply to the overwhelming majority of great golfers who ever lived.

Fundamental No. 1:
Balanced Address Position

The first thing that good players do in their golf swing is address the ball in balance. There are many different definitions of balance. I've heard teachers say that you have to have the weight on the heels, or drop the right shoulder

Fig. 3.1 Balanced address position

and tilt the spine to the right. But there are really just two important aspects to determine if a player is in balance in the address position.

1. The weight should be evenly divided on both feet, with the majority of the weight directly under the arches of the feet *(Fig. 3.1)*.

2. The hip joint should stack directly above the ankle joint *(Fig. 3.2)*. If these two joints aren't aligned, the body is out of balance, pure and simple *(Fig. 3.3)*.

Notice in *Fig. 3.2* that the kneecaps are over the shoelaces, the shoulders are just outside the toes, and the ear is aligned with the spine down to the hip joint. The majority of the weight is directly on the arches of the feet.

Every sport, including golf, is played in balance, with the balls of the feet providing much of the support. Biomechanical research has proven this. In Chapter 4, we'll explain why. The old notion that the weight should be dominantly on the heels contradicts basic laws of balance. Some golfers have started out on their heels in the address position, but their weight quickly moved forward into the middle of the foot as they went into their forward press. Nancy Lopez is a great example of this. Early in her career, when she addressed the

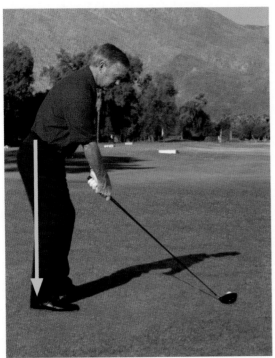

Fig. 3.2 Balanced address: Notice how the hip joint stacks on top of the ankle.

Fig. 3.3 Out of balance: The hip joint is splayed outside the ankle, indicating that the weight is on the heels.

Fig. 3.4 The left side of the upper torso shifts the weight immediately to the right side.

ball, her weight was on her heels. However, she began her forward press by raising her hands, and as she did so, her weight would come off her heels and onto her arches into a neutral balanced position. If the weight remains on the heels, it is anatomically impossible to shift the weight effectively with the feet throughout the swing. If the weight should remain on the heels, as many people have advocated, then why is it that skilled players always rise up off of their heels as they swing through the shot?

At this point I want to make an observation: We have been told that the hips and shoulders should always be parallel to the line of flight. (Think of the old railroad tracks image, with the line of the feet, knees, hips, and shoulders as the inner rail and the clubhead line as the outer rail.) Although this is pretty much true, the reality is that if you watch Tour players, you'll notice that their shoulders are slightly rotated and aimed to the left of the target line anywhere from 0 to 17 degrees. The range for their hips varies from around 2 degrees closed to 6 degrees open. This is due to the fact that they have the right hand below the left hand when they grip the club. This subtle extension of the right arm forces the right shoulder to protrude slightly forward, which then has the shoulders aiming *slightly* left. As a person gets older and develops rounded and rotated shoulders, this becomes a problem because the increased rotation of the shoulders will encourage an over-the-top move.

From a neutral address position, the golfer should feel light and can move easily into the second fundamental.

Fundamental No. 2: **Early Weight Transfer**

Computer analysis shows that the best players shift approximately 70 percent of their weight onto their right foot before the club is even a few feet away from the ball. What's fascinating about this move is that there are so many different ways to do it. Gary Player, Arnold Palmer, and Vijay Singh kick their right knee in and then rebound. Jack Nicklaus has a very slight press with his body into his left side as he cocks his head to the right. After slightly pressing into his left side, Nicklaus then pushes the shaft back with his left shoulder as he moves deep into his right side. Nicklaus

Fig. 3.5 A loaded right hip and braced lower body allow the spine to angle slightly to the right, creating the V.

their knees and then rebound. Julius Boros and Bruce Summerhays bounced the club on the ground before initiating the swing, as does Fuzzy Zoeller. Whatever the method, the actual backswing starts with a tension release in which the energy slightly pushes into the left side and then is released and flows into the right side.

When I say "flows into the right side," I'm referring not only to the weight moving onto the right foot, but also into the muscles of the right leg, and especially the right hip, which goes into a state of contraction and becomes "loaded." Loading the right hip properly is arguably the most important aspect of the backswing *(Fig. 3.5)*. If the hip is not fully coiled, the upper body inevitably takes control and begins the downswing process.

Common examples of not loading the hips properly are sliding *(Fig. 3.6)*, overturning *(Fig. 3.7)*, and elevating the rear hip by straightening the leg *(Fig. 3.8)*. Keeping the right hip stable

has described this as a rebounding off of his left side.

Most players forward press with their hands, or even change pressure in their hands, followed by a rebound. Golfers such as Nick Faldo, Tom Kite, and Curtis Strange bump or squat with

Fig. 3.6 Hip slide

Fig. 3.7 Overturning of hips

Fig. 3.8 Elevated hip due to straightening of the leg

Fig. 3.9 The majority of the shoulder turn has taken place when the left arm is parallel to the ground.

Fig. 3.10 There is not much difference in shoulder rotation at the top of the backswing than where they were half way back.

gives you the best shot at having it unwind in proper sequence on the downswing.

At the halfway-back position (my definition of halfway back is when the left arm is parallel to the ground), we'll see a slight head movement to the right, with the right shoulder deeply turned. We'll also see how the left shoulder has moved away from the left side, which forms the letter V, or a hypotenuse triangle *(Fig. 3.5)*, a very common position on a full swing. It is also important to notice how the left shoulder has moved past the left hip and behind the left knee. If we draw a diagonal line across the shoulders at the halfway-back position, we'll notice that most good players have turned their shoulders approximately 60 to 70 degrees *(Fig. 3.9)*. Some, such as Vijay

Singh and Arnold Palmer, turn them closer to 90 degrees.

If we compare their shoulder turn at the halfway-back position to where they are at the completion of the backswing *(Fig. 3.10)*, we see that there isn't that much difference. In other words, most of the shoulder turn is accomplished early in the swing.

To make this point even more clearly, the weight that I'm referring to is actually the upper-body weight of the left side. In other words, good players turn and shift their upper torso early and deeply into the backswing against the resistance of the lower body. The more a golfer turns his shoulders against the bracing of the legs, the more torque he creates in his body. The bracing of the legs is absolutely crucial, because if there is a caving in of any kind with the lower body, the stretch and torque will be lost. Loss of stability in the backswing is most commonly due to (1) sliding the hips and having too much of a bend in the left knee, (2) elevating the hip due to straightening the right leg, which usually forces the upper torso to lift, or (3) overturning the hips, which forces the weight to go to the outside of the right foot. To better picture this, imagine you're going to shoot a rubber band across the room by placing it around your left forefinger. The forefinger represents your left leg and left hip. The rubber band represents the left shoulder and lats. As you pull the rubber band back with the fingers of your right hand, the more you keep the left finger stable, the more power you'll generate out of the rubber band. If, however, you move the left finger back toward the right-hand fingers, you'll lose all of the energy that you're trying to store up. This stretching is absolutely crucial throughout the golf swing.

Creating separation between the lower body and upper body is crucial for generating torque between the two body halves and makes it considerably easier for the right hip to begin pushing off to start the downswing, immediately followed by the left-side muscles pulling the torso into the left side. If these muscles aren't loaded properly, the start of the downswing will almost certainly begin with an improper sequencing. This is precisely what we're going to talk about in fundamental number 3.

Fundamental No. 3: **Transition into the Forward Swing: Face-On View**

As the lower body is unwinding *first* during the transition, the left knee will plant itself on top of the ball of the left foot *(Fig. 3.12)*. This move is the make-or-break point in the entire downswing. When the left knee plants itself on top of the left foot, the dynamic force of the weight shift sends a shock wave up the femur, and in a millisecond, dramatically forces the left hip to begin clearing.

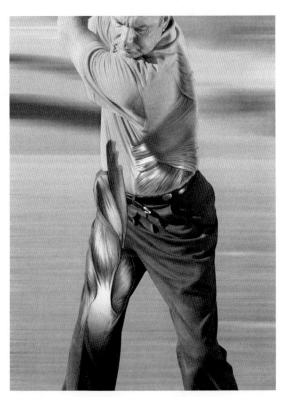

Fig. 3.11 An illustration of the right-side muscles contracting and the left side expanding, all ready to release.

Fig. 3.12 The lateral/rotational shift of the hips must start the downswing.

This move is clearly visible when track-and-field athletes throw a discus or hammer. The more powerfully they land on the front foot and leg, the more effective they are in hurling the object. If the left knee doesn't move back and put weight on the left foot, the golfer does not benefit from the power that he has generated and stored up in the backswing. There is no clear-cut stop at the top of the backswing with all of the body parts. In other words, as the left knee is pulling back, we actually see an increased separation between the left and right legs going forward *(Fig. 3.13)*. This increased separation creates more power and consistency in the swing.

The shifting of the lower body actually increases the stretch between the lower body and the upper torso. This is the same kind of movement as hitting a baseball or a tennis ball. Watch a baseball batter as he waits for the pitcher to deliver a pitch. Once he picks up the pitch, he strides and steps into the ball. His left leg begins the separation, but the bat still hasn't swung forward. This is the same sequence as the golf swing and is the most important move in the golf swing motion. At this point, the lower body actually accelerates into the left side, but once it gets there, the hips brake, and a millisecond after that, the upper trunk moves and brakes, then the arms, then

Fig. 3.13 Notice how Tom Kite's hips shift powerfully over onto his left foot.

the club. These forces hit the left leg, creating a shock wave up the femur, which then forces the left hip to rotate and create what I call the "two-cheek position" (see page 35). It's important to have a stable lower body, because without the solid base in control, the upper body nearly always starts the downswing first, creating a loss of power and direction into the motion.

A moment after the ball is struck, the body and hands release. Somewhere between impact and when the right arm is parallel to the ground on the follow-through, we should see three fingers (the little, ring, and middle fingers) of the left-hand glove under the right

wrist *(Fig. 3.14)*. This indicates that the club has been released. This position is a result of the centrifugal force created by the turning of the left hip and shoulder, which allows the club to continue to accelerate as the arms and wrists to begin the journey upward into the follow-through.

The overwhelming majority of high handicappers either (1) don't release the club and hold on *(Fig. 3.15)* or (2) uncock the wrists too early in the downswing. A proper release occurs when the sequencing of the body parts shift onto the left leg and the timing of the arms and hands follows. There has been much controversy about what creates a proper release. Many teachers believe that the release is created by a conscious swinging of the arms and hands; others believe that the release is a natural by-product of the body shifting and rotating properly. I tend to agree with the latter, mainly because I've asked countless great players with great hand action what they feel with their hands, and to this day, none of them have told me that they're conscious about what their hands are doing through impact. Also, when people try to manipulate their hands and arms into the downswing, whether they know it or not, they often add pressure and tension to their arms, which slows down the body speed. However, I've also seen students who, once they became conscious of releasing the club with their hands, were actually able to control the sequencing of their arms with their body.

Generally speaking, with good players, I tend to work with their bodies more, and with high handicappers, I try to get them to feel their arms and club more. In any case, the club must be released.

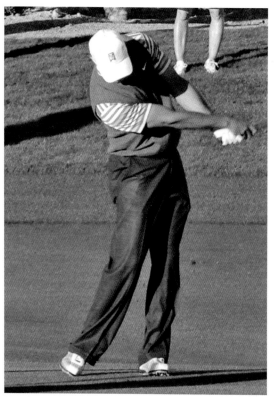

Fig. 3.14 Tiger Woods releasing after impact, with three fingers of the left-hand glove clearly visible under the right wrist.

Fig. 3.15 Notice the position of the golfer's glove above the right arm, indicating no release.

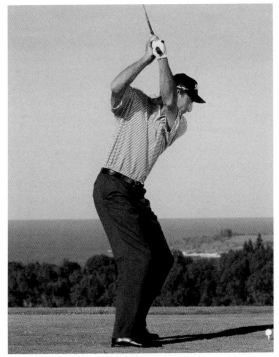

Fig. 3.16 Jim Furyk's upright swing plane

Fig. 3.17 Sergio Garcia with a laid-off shaft

Transition into the Forward Swing:
Down-The-Line View

Viewing the transition from the down-the-line view is even more revealing. At the top of the backswing, we see players in a wide variety of positions. We've seen great players with upright swing planes *(Fig. 3.16)*, laid-off planes *(Fig. 3.17)*, and neutral planes. We've seen great

players with cupped wrists like Freddie Couples *(Fig. 3.18)*, flat wrists like Jack Nicklaus *(Fig. 3.19)*, and convex wrists like Lee Trevino and especially Dustin Johnson *(Fig. 3.20)*. Great players have played from all of these positions.

No matter where great players are at the top of their backswing, once they initiate the downswing by unwinding their hips, the arms

Fig. 3.18 Freddie Couples's cupped wrists

Fig. 3.19 Jack Nicklaus's flat wrists

Fig. 3.20 Dustin Johnson's convex wrists

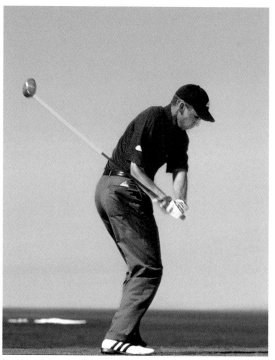

Fig. 3.21 The lateral shift of the hips drops the shaft under the right shoulder and above the right hip.

and shaft will drop and come into the ball from a point between their right hip and their right shoulder *(Fig. 3.21)*. The shaft must come into the ball from behind the ball, not on top of it. Again, it is the unwinding of the hips that creates this position. Unfortunately, the vast majority of high handicappers bring the club into the ball from outside, or above, the right shoulder *(Fig. 3.22)*. This is commonly known as "coming over the top" and is caused by the upper body, rather than the lower body, starting the downswing. The over-the-top move is normally a symptom of the right hip not being loaded properly on the backswing, which in turn forces the upper body and arms to get out of proper sequence and start the downswing.

Fig. 3.22 A classic over-the-top move

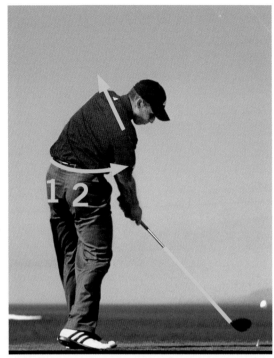

Fig. 3.23 Both cheeks of the fanny are clearly visible in these—and all—great players at the point of impact.

THE TWO-CHEEK POSITION

As I mentioned earlier, every Tour player arrives at impact in what I call the two-cheek position *(Fig. 3.23)*. From the down-the-line view, we can see both cheeks of the fanny, the left shoulder aimed slightly to the left, and the right heel off the ground. They are all in this position without exception—some more so than others.

The vast majority of high handicappers arrive at impact with one or no cheeks showing *(Fig. 3.24)*, with little or no shoulder rotation, and with no weight off the right foot.

Immediately after impact, the club disappears from view because the player's body is in the way of the camera. When the club reappears, we want to see it under the left shoulder *(Fig. 3.25)*. This is on a similar path that the

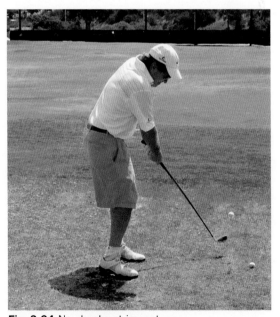

Fig. 3.24 No cheeks at impact

Fig. 3.25 Correct: The shaft reappears at a point between the left hip and left shoulder on a similar path that was traveled on the downswing, where the shaft bisected the right shoulder and right hip.

Fig. 3.26 Incorrect: The shaft reappears too high.

club was on as it started the downswing. With the vast majority of high handicappers, the shaft reappears above the left shoulder *(Fig. 3.26)*. If the lower body shifts as it should on the downswing, it will rotate. When it rotates, the club will go to the inside. The club should then finish high but high to the left—fully rotated to the inside, not going down the target line. From here, the club will finish around and behind the golfer's head in what I call the "Steve Martin look." If you recall, when Steve Martin began his standup comedy routine, he would walk onstage with the old arrow-through-the-head prop. The shaft should bisect your head, just like an arrow going through it *(Figs. 3.27 and 3.28)*. Just getting into this position cures a lot of swing faults.

In essence, the anatomical function of one's body dictates the golf swing motion, and the golf swing motion creates the swing mechanics, not the other way around.

Remember the three fundamentals:

1. A neutral, balanced stance

2. An early weight transfer into the right side

3. A transition of the weight to the left side and into the two-cheek position and finish

Perhaps the biggest problem in golf today, even among some very good players, is that so many players don't transfer their weight onto their left foot on the forward swing. Weight transfer is the shifting of the upper torso into the right hip and side on the backswing, and the unwinding of the right hip working in unison with the pulling of the left side on the downswing. Incorporated in this process is good balance, because the swing will seldom ever be effective without it. I cannot emphasize enough that the nucleus of the swing is the body, and how well we train it to be flexible and strong will enable it to move with ease.

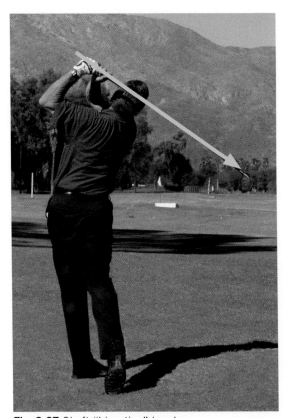

Fig. 3.27 Shaft "bisecting" head

Fig. 3.28 Shaft "bisecting" head

Fig. 3.29 Jamie Sadlowski, 2008 & 2009 RE/MAX World Long Drive champion

Fig. 3.30 John Daly, one of the PGA Tour's longest drivers

DIFFERENT BODY TYPES, SAME FLEXIBILITY

Many people say Tiger Woods has the perfect body type for golf. I don't know about that. Jack Nicklaus isn't built like Woods, and he did pretty well. And Arnold Palmer isn't built like either one of them. Flexibility and strength come in all kinds of packages. One body is not necessarily better than another when it comes to golf.

The common factors among all good golfers are efficient mobility and stability, which lead to a balanced golf swing. Add power, and what you have is an unbeatable combination as demonstrated by Jamie Sadlowski and John Daly, who each have different body types and superb flexibility (Figs. 3.29 and 3.30).

CHAPTER 4

WHAT THE MUSCLES
DO IN THE GOLF SWING

WHAT EXACTLY IS A GOLF SWING? The golf swing is a motion performed by the body, which in turn swings the golf club. Since the body is composed of hundreds of muscles, all of which are designed to move and/or stabilize bones and joints, the relationship between the muscles and the golf swing should be obvious: How well the muscles function and interact with each other determines how well the body swings the club. In other words, golf swing mechanics are really indicators of how the muscles move and interact with one another in this kinetic chain.

In addition, golfers who have strong, flexible, and functional muscles are able to perform this motion much easier than golfers with weak and tight muscles. After all, a younger, athletic person, in most cases, has a much easier time hitting a golf ball, tennis ball, or baseball than a senior citizen whose muscles have become tighter and weaker.

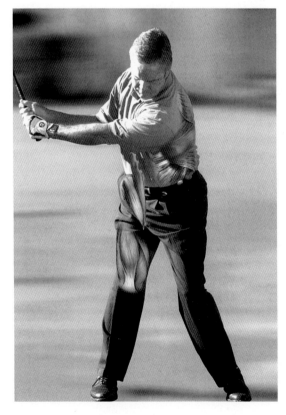

The good news is that no one has to take a course in physical education or anatomy to get an understanding of how the muscles affect the golf swing. However, some basic knowledge is helpful. The Creator designed the muscles of the body to work synergically. When the muscles function according to their design, we attain perfect posture, and the muscles move our joints in the manner in which they were designed—that is, to move within our environment. These 650-plus muscles all have a specific purpose, or as I like to say, they all have a job to perform. Let's take a look at the role the muscles play in the body and how they work in the golf swing.

Fig. 4.1 A neutral position

Biceps Contracting

Triceps Expanding

Fig. 4.2 An example of how the muscles work together

HOW MUSCLES WORK

Muscles work in pairs. For example, in our upper arms are the biceps. On the underside of the upper arms are the triceps. When the biceps contract, the triceps expand and vice versa (*Figs. 4.1 and 4.2*). This phenomenon is called reciprocal inhibition. It is simply the means by which muscles interact with each other.

Another example of how the muscles interact is exhibited by lifting a heavy suitcase up to your chest and into the trunk of your car. As you begin the lift, a little muscle called the supraspinatus engages and enlists its help to the hand and arm. As the supraspinatus begins contracting, it cries out to the deltoid for help, which then assists in the process. Finally, as the suitcase gets higher, the deltoid cries out for help and then asks the rhomboids and trapezii (traps) to help, and now you've got the suitcase up and into the trunk. There is a chain reaction

of all of the muscles working together. If one or more of the muscles is weak or dysfunctional, additional stress and pressure is transferred to another muscle. This kinematic sequencing is the same way the muscles work throughout the golf swing—or any other athletic motion for that matter.

THE MUSCULATURE OF THE BODY

In the front of our bodies, starting with our lower legs, we have the front of the calves (tibialis anterior), the quadriceps (quads), the hip flexors, the abdominals, and the pectorals *(Fig. 4.3)*. They reciprocate with the backs of the calves (soleus and gastrocnemius), the hamstrings, the glutes, the lower-back muscles, and the upper-back muscles (rhomboids, trapezii, lats, and so forth) *(Fig. 4.4)*.

Let's take a look at the primary hip flexor (iliopsoas), which is a very powerful muscle in our body. The iliopsoas plays a vital role because it attaches onto three bones—the femur, pelvis, and spine. It also has a major effect on the diaphragm and sympathetic nervous system. When the hip flexors become imbalanced (usually when one side becomes stronger and tighter than the other), every single joint in the body is affected. The maintenance of the iliopsoas is crucial to posture, the golf swing, and all sports activity.

Deltoids
Pectorals
Biceps
Abdominals
Hips-Psoas, Iliacus
Abductor
Quadriceps
Tibialis Anterior

Fig. 4.3 Anterior (front) muscle groups

Rhomboids, Trapezius
Triceps
Erectors
Hip Rotators
Glutes
Hamstrings
Gastrocnemius/ Soleus

Fig. 4.4 Posterior (back) muscle groups

THE MUSCLES
IN THE ADDRESS POSITION

Once we assume the address position, the front muscles begin to contract and the back muscles expand *(Fig. 4.5)*. As we tilt forward from our hips, our center of gravity comes outside the body and relocates a few inches in front of our hips. When our muscles work properly during the golf swing, they protect this center of gravity and help us remain balanced. The end result is more solid and consistent contact.

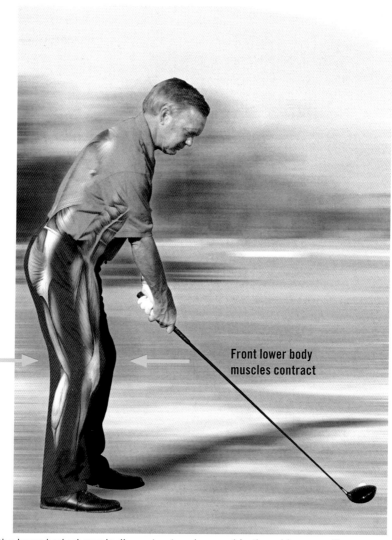

Back lower body muscles expand

Front lower body muscles contract

Fig. 4.5 Muscles of the lower body dynamically contract and expand in the address position.

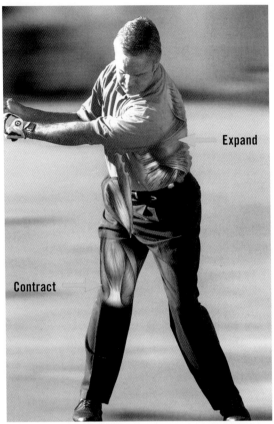

Fig. 4.6 Lower-body muscles on the front of the right leg and hip contract and left-side muscles of the upper torso expand in the backswing.

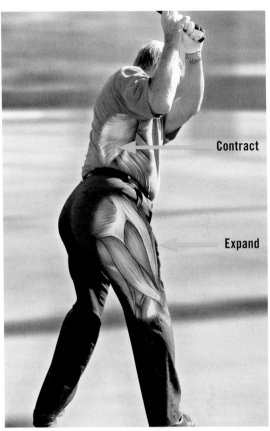

Fig. 4.7 Muscles on the back of the right leg expand and right-side muscles of the upper torso contract in the backswing.

THE BACKSWING

Now the action begins. As the left side of the upper torso shifts into the right side, the center of gravity moves slightly to the right. The front lower-body muscles, calves, quads, and hip flexors contract *(Fig. 4.6)*. (Just as the biceps do in the illustration.) As these muscles contract, the muscles in the back of the lower body (calves, hamstrings, and glutes) expand

(Fig. 4.7). Holding all of this together are the quads and hip flexors working in conjunction with the glutes in stabilizing the lower body. As the front and back of the body are conducting this tug-of-war, the lower half and upper half of the body are having their own battle. That is, the front of the chest (the pecs) expands *(Fig. 4.8)*, while the upper muscles of the back (rhomboids and traps) contract

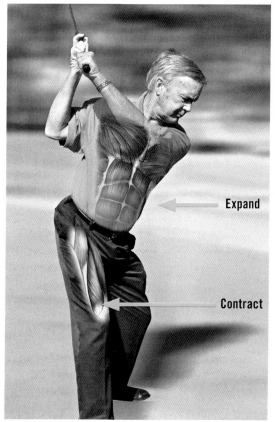

Expand

Contract

Fig. 4.8 Chest muscles expand and quadriceps and hip contract in the backswing.

Contract

Expand

Fig. 4.9 Back muscles contract and hamstrings expand in the backswing.

(Fig. 4.9). The front lower-body muscles contract while the chest muscles expand. The lower posterior muscles of the legs expand, and the upper-back muscles (rhomboids and traps) contract.

Tightened and shortened muscles on the front side of our chests normally pull the shoulders forward with them, creating rounded shoulders. Rounded shoulders have a damaging effect on the expansion of the chest throughout the golf swing and will definitely produce a restricted shoulder turn and a myriad of other swing faults.

If that's not enough, the right and left sides of the body are also fighting each other. While the right-side muscles contract, the left-side muscles expand. In effect, there are three simultaneous battles going on: (1) upper-body versus lower-body muscles, (2) front versus back muscles, and (3) right-side versus left-side muscles. In the midst of these battles, all of the muscles are trying to keep the center of gravity in balance.

THE MOST IMPORTANT MOVE
The Transition at the Start of the Downswing

I, like virtually every golf instructor, have been asked many times, "What actually starts the downswing?" The reality is I've asked the same question to many of golf's greatest players, and I've gotten a lot of different answers. No matter what these great players feel, there is definitely a sequence that does occur in all of their golf swings. Let's take a look at what physiologically happens from a musculoskeletal point of view.

The powerful hip flexor in the right hip is wound up because it holds all of these muscle battles together *(Fig. 4.10)*. It is being loaded, twisted, and contorted, and it definitely wants to get out of there, so it immediately begins to unwind itself. As it pushes off, it works in unison with the left hip and leg, and the weight then begins to transfer over to the left side. In a millisecond, with all this unwinding, the center of gravity moves back toward the front foot. As the weight shifts onto the left side, the muscles of the left leg begin to contract *(Fig. 4.11)* and do precisely what the right side muscles were doing on the backswing. In other words, as the weight shifts and crashes onto the left foot, a shock wave is created that races up the leg and puts pressure on the head of the left femur and

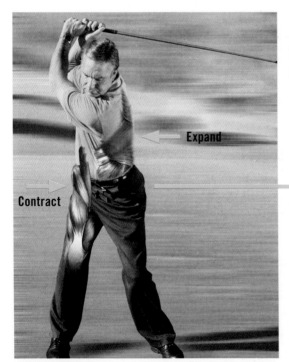

Fig. 4.10 The right hip and leg muscles push off in the downswing.

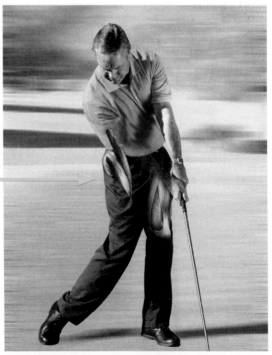

Fig. 4.11 The left hip and leg muscles pull in the downswing.

left hip. These forces then cause the left hip to clear out of the way. This in turn releases the upper trunk. Next the arms are released, followed by the uncocking of the wrists.

This is how it works in the golf swing and in other athletic motions as well. As you can see, an effective golf swing requires quite a lot of coordinated interaction of the muscles throughout the body, especially in the legs and hips. For example, strong and functional legs provide a great foundation on which the upper body can twist and turn. If a person has tight hamstrings or weak quads, the hamstrings and quads will not be able to accept the tremendous forces placed upon them. The legs will usually

straighten up, causing a laying off and then a lifting of the club. The hamstrings are also connected to a little ring around the pelvis called the ischial tuberosity, so they directly affect the stabilization and rotation of the hips, which affects the center of gravity.

When stabilization of the legs and hips is lost, the upper body will normally compensate and begin to take over the golf swing motion *(Fig. 4.12)*. In addition to the club being pulled to the inside, the straightening of the leg will normally cause the shoulders to flatten, affecting the hand and club position. This will usually cause an over-the-top move, simply because the lower body has lost control.

Fig. 4.12 Failure to properly load the right hip in the backswing makes it nearly impossible to produce an effective transition into the ball.

To illustrate this more clearly, imagine a quarterback going back to pass. On this particular play, as he drops back and plants his rear foot, a defensive lineman grabs a hold of his lower body in an attempt to bring him down. With his legs now in the grasp of the tackler, the QB is stuck and can't shift his weight. He is left with only relying on a flailing motion with his hands and arms to throw the ball.

Many teachers who see this prescribe a cure for the over-the-top move, but in reality it is a symptom of lower-body dysfunction (the straightening of the legs). Another typical example is a person with quads and hips that are too tight or overdeveloped. We see this typically in skiers, bicyclists, marathoners, and bodybuilders. These athletes tend to get out of balance in their legs, a by-product of overtraining their quads and hip flexors. The overtrained, overdeveloped muscles become shortened, which then causes them to lose their rotational capacity. This lack of flexibility and rotational capacity generally causes a sliding of the hips out to the right, which results in an upper-body reverse spine angle, and often a chicken wing. This makes it impossible to get the upper body behind the left leg or to get the club properly behind one's shoulders.

Another glaring physical dysfunction is an inflexible torso. (Remember that PGA Tour players have 50 to 100 percent more flexibility in their upper trunks than the average person.) When a person with limited mobility in the upper trunk tries to make a full shoulder turn and can't do it, compensations will almost inevitably occur, and they can include any or all of the following: lifting, collapsed arms, flattening of the shoulders, and, most harmful,

losing lower-body stability. In short, the synchronicity (or kinematic sequence) of the muscle chains is lost. They no longer work together, resulting in a jerky and choppy motion in the swing. People who have tight lats and tight and overdeveloped pecs (bodybuilders, for example) usually have severely bent arms at the top of their backswings. Remember that the pec muscles must expand on the backswing. If a person has tight pecs or lats, the shoulders simply can't rotate effectively throughout the swing. The rotation of the trunk creates extension of the arms, and tight trunk muscles usually restrict extension, hence chicken wings.

GOLFERS ARE ATHLETES

Swinging a golf club is a tremendously energetic, athletic movement. It is no wonder that so many people can't do it effectively. Their bodies do not possess the strength or flexibility in the major muscle groups to perform this highly skilled gymnastic activity. This is why just working on your golf swing mechanics is not necessarily going to make your body stronger and more flexible. Practice alone is not enough to allow you to discover or regain a fountain of youth. I advocate a deeper look and new perspective on the golf swing. Rather than just working on your swing mechanics, first examine how your muscles are affecting your mechanics. Again, your body *is* your golf swing. Improving the function of your muscles will obviously improve the function of your golf swing, but not necessarily the other way around. For most golfers, this new perspective is a must. But fear not. In the next few chapters, I will show you how you can get your muscles to begin moving as they were designed to move. You can create a freer and more powerful golf swing. You can enhance your enjoyment of the greatest game mankind has ever devised, and it can last a lifetime.

RESEARCH STUDIES: WHY TOURING PROS ARE MORE FLEXIBLE

In the early 1980s, several research studies provided an entirely new perspective on the golf swing. A significant study was conducted by the biomechanics laboratory at Centinela Hospital Medical Center in Inglewood, California. Around the same time, renowned biomechanics pioneer Dr. Gideon Ariel and physical therapists Ric McDonald and Pete Egoscue were conducting their own studies. Among other results, the study by Centinela Hospital showed

Fig. 4.13 David Duval demonstrating superb upper-torso flexibility

that PGA Tour players have an average of 50 to 100 percent more flexibility in their upper trunks than the average person *(Fig. 4.13)*. Incredibly, the study showed they had even more flexibility on average than NBA basketball players! In addition, PGA Tour players had about two-thirds faster hip speed in their forward swings than the average golfer.

There was some question about why these professional golfers possessed this physical advantage until the researchers realized that the answer was because they all started the game when they were kids. When you consider how gymnastic the turning of the hips and shoulders are in the golf swing, and that most pros have been performing this motion hundreds of times a day for a lifetime, their superb upper-body flexibility is no mystery.

But how about hip speed? That's simple. Hip speed is a function of how well the leg muscles support and drive the hips. A round of golf is a 5- to 7-mile walk, and these pros play and practice nearly every day. They walk, or are on their feet, for much of their lives. Subsequently, they end up with incredibly powerful legs, floating hips, and superb upper-body flexibility.

Because the average golfer hasn't been out there turning his body and walking as much as these Tour players, and instead has been sitting at a desk or driving a car, it's easy to understand why he ends up with weaker legs, tighter hips, and a tighter trunk. It's no wonder that so many can't adequately perform a fundamental golf swing.

CHAPTER 5

YOU'VE GOT TO BE HIP

AS WE'VE DISCUSSED, the hips play a vital role in the human body. They are the bridge between the lower and upper torso. They dictate posture and play a major role in both a person's anatomical function and athletic performance. Even the slightest alteration of the hip joints can affect every other joint in the body. For example, if the pelvis is pulled too far forward due to an overtightening and shortening of the hip muscles (which occurs in the overwhelming majority of people in our culture), the muscles along the lower lumbar can be stressed to such an extent that they pull the spine out of position (hello, back pain). In addition to an excessive forward anterior tilt of the pelvis, most people have one side that is usually tighter than the other, which forces the hips to also be rotated *(Fig. 5.1)*.

This was certainly the case with me back in my younger days, as my hips were not only severely anteriorly tilted but also severely rotated to the left due to the dominance of my right hip. The severe rotation of my hips to the left forced my left foot to flare outward, creating what's called tibial and femoral torsion (this means that my tibia and femur were going in different directions). With my left hip and left knee rotated outward and turned to the left, a tremendous force was placed on the inside of that knee. This was the cause of my knee pain (and subsequent surgeries). Today, I realize that I could have had 10 more surgeries that wouldn't have been effective, because only when I straightened out my hips did I realign the hip-knee-ankle relationship. To summarize, it was the misalignment of my hips that caused my knee problems, not the

Fig. 5.1 A classic example of tight hips pulling the shoulders and head forward

Fig. 5.2 Weak hips creating a C-curve posture (flat back). This posture type indicates weakness.

Fig. 5.3 A tight and dominate right hip tends to pull the right shoulder down and rotate it to the left.

knee itself. In other words, the knee was the scene of the crime, not the cause of it.

My experience has taught me that the misalignment of the hips is responsible for the vast majority of joint and musculoskeletal problems. Only when the hips return to their proper anatomical position can the body's other joints be restored to their correct anatomical position with no undue stress or friction. The misalignment of my hips was also the primary cause of the deterioration of my golf swing and golf game. When my hips were rotated to the left and my right hip and right shoulder were pulled forward, they hindered my ability to turn my right shoulder behind me in the backswing. This also caused my hip and shoulder plane to flatten out and prevented me from having enough side bend.

With my shoulders and hips on a flat plane, *(Fig. 5.2)* my hips were encouraged to spin out on the forward swing (or, as they say in baseball, "step in the bucket"). The spinout made it nearly impossible to shift my weight onto the forward foot and have my left knee align on top of my left foot. Not only could I not make an efficient weight transfer, but this put a tremendous amount of stress on my left knee and ankle, and in time, I began to wear down the ligaments and cartilage in my knee.

A true weight transfer is where the left hip is over the left knee, which is over the left foot. When these joints on the left side stack up at impact, a shock wave is produced from the ground and up the femur, forcing the left hip to clear and create clubhead speed and power in the shot. The inability to generate rotational speed around the left hip and leg results in a loss of power, and it forces the golfer to compensate in other ways, usually by flipping the hands.

The misalignment of the hips *(Fig. 5.3)* (usually due to the dominance of the right hip, for right-handers) is really the genesis of most swing faults and the number one cause of poor golf shots. Having said that, do you remember what controls bones? Muscles. Restoring function to the muscles restores function to the bones, which restores function to the golf swing motion. The critical nature of the hips in the golf swing cannot be overstated. The function of the right hip (for right-handers) is the single most important factor in the golf swing. All my research and experience gathered over 4 decades leads me to believe that the golfer's most common problem is tight and imbalanced hips.

Let's take a look at the role the hips play throughout the swing. In a true weight transfer, the right hip engages on the backswing due to the left-side upper-body weight being shifted upon it. These forces placed upon the hip joint then force the head of the femur to rotate in its socket, which forces the shoulders to turn. Starting down, the unwinding of the right hip (generated by the muscles) forces the hips to shift back to the left. This is the make-or-break point in the golf swing. It is here where the result of the shot is determined. In this millisecond, the left hip joint must line up right above the left knee, which must stack up over the ball of the left foot. If this doesn't happen, the golfer sacrifices control of the clubhead.

STACKING UP

As you can see, the joints of the body are designed to stack up, or align right on top of each other. They are always seeking that posi-

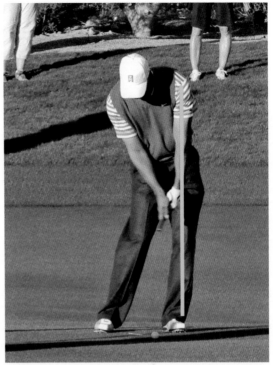

Fig. 5.4 Left shoulder, hip, knee, and foot perfectly stacked up

tion. Try jumping off a chair and landing on the floor. Your feet will always come down pointing straight ahead with the knees and hips lined up right above them. In my postaccident swings, my misaligned joints caused not only my injuries but also my golf swing faults. Nearly everything in my teaching is geared to getting the body functioning so that the joints are in proper alignment. At impact on an iron, the left shoulder, hip, knee, and foot should line up *(Fig. 5.4)*. Keep in mind that the left hip will be turned, as will the left shoulder. They are not lined up linearly or vertically, because the left hip has rotated. A driver is somewhat different because we hit up on it, and as a result, we're somewhat more behind the ball than on an iron.

CENTER OF GRAVITY MOVEMENT

The secret to virtually every sport is protecting the center of gravity (COG), or balance. In a balanced body, the joints line up properly and, as a result, they function the way they were designed to function. Keeping the COG balanced also helps eliminate tension.

This is crucial because tension is public enemy number one when it comes to performing a smooth golf swing. A body free of tension allows the body and mind to function smoothly and efficiently. Deep within our bodies we have a center. This center is contained in the very middle of our weight, at a point approximately 1 inch below our navels and 1 inch in. This is

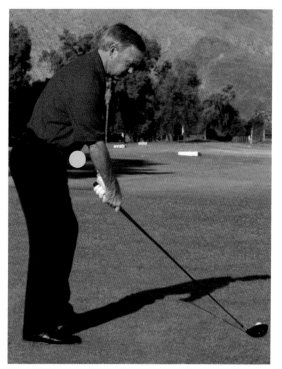

Fig. 5.5 Center of gravity moves slightly out of the address position

the center of gravity, which controls all of our balanced movements.

Watch a tightrope walker on a high wire: With every centimeter that he moves off balance, the balance pole counters this, helping recenter him. In the golf swing, the golf club reacts much like the balance pole. Research shows that for every centimeter the center of gravity moves during the golf swing, the clubhead can fluctuate up to 14 inches out of its orbit. In other words, the more the COG moves, the more compensation the golfer needs to make in the swing.

In the golf swing, once we bend from the hips in the address position, the COG moves just outside and in front of the body, still in front and slightly below the navel *(Fig. 5.5)*. Keeping this point quiet is a key factor in the golf swing (from a physics point of view) and directly affects the quality of any golf shot.

I used to study center of gravity movement on the computers designed by Dr. Gideon Ariel, one of the true pioneers of computerized biomechanics. I was fascinated by Edwin Moses, the most acclaimed high hurdler of all time. Dr. Ariel's computers were able to measure Moses's COG as he jumped over the 42-inch-high hurdles. The amazing thing was that his COG hardly fluctuated at all. This is what really separated Moses from other hurdlers, whose COG moved up and down too much. We see this same type of fluctuation in the COG with high handicappers: The more lifting, sliding, and overall excess movements they perform, the more their COG is compromised. When the COG is jumping all over the place, energy is lost. Of course, the COG does not stay completely still during the golf swing. Why? We

Fig. 5.6 COG in neutral

Fig. 5.7 COG moves slightly over to the right hip

Fig. 5.8 COG moves forward to the point where the left hip was in the address position

have two pivot points: a right hip and a left hip. For this reason, the golf swing is not a true circle (as was once believed and taught) but more of an elliptical arc.

Although our goal is to keep the COG from moving excessively, it must move somewhat to accommodate the shifting of the weight—a little to the right then back a little to the left and then back toward the left heel *(Figs. 5.6–5.8)*. We certainly don't want it to move up and down, although some players do lower the COG slightly as they drop down into a shot. This is very common among successful players, with Tiger Woods and Byron Nelson being great examples. However, the players that do drop down into the shot usually stand in a more upright manner in the address position. Golfers who squat or sit low at address have a harder time staying level and usually tend to lift

up on the backswing and in the downswing. It's much better to drop down than to lift up. When golfers lift up through the shot, they almost invariably lose their lag and their control of the club. This is power leakage. As the body and COG go up, the club is forced down. We want to store up energy for as long as possible, not prematurely release it.

With the COG in the proper position, the muscles stay contracted during the downswing, keeping the energy locked in and the wrists cocked for as long as possible. This is a result of the forces of gravity and muscle contraction that are being placed on the body, which then rush out through the club.

How do we keep the COG in the proper position throughout the golf swing? The answer is simple: strong and flexible legs and hips (and a strong and flexible upper body doesn't hurt, either). Weak and unstable legs and hips will not provide the stability the upper body and arms desperately need to achieve maximum coil and torque, not to mention balance and power.

There is much talk that the lower body isn't that important in the golf swing. Teachers who say this attempt to prove the theory by getting down on their knees and hitting powerful golf shots. The next time you see this, take a look at their hips while they're swinging on their knees. You will see their hips rotate quite powerfully and their knees digging into the ground. If these people hit a golf ball while sitting on a table with their feet off the ground, the results would not be the same. Stability with the ground is a paramount fundamental of every active sport.

Let's get back to center of gravity. If the COG rises up on the backswing, you will see a lifting of the club, which takes the lower-body muscles out of contraction *(Figs. 5.9 and 5.10).* In other words, the body's muscles will be unloaded in an unproductive move, shifted back on the heels during the backswing. Both scenarios usually result from straightening the right leg, preventing the proper loading of the right hip. On the downswing, we frequently see the COG raising because of the lower-body muscles not firing, usually because they were not loaded on the backswing. (After all, you can't unload something that hasn't been loaded). In this case, the muscles have been taken out of contraction (shown by the lack of the flex in the knees), which then impedes a dynamic move into the ball.

Protecting the COG is crucial in the golf swing, and the way to protect it from moving too much is by possessing strength and flexibil-

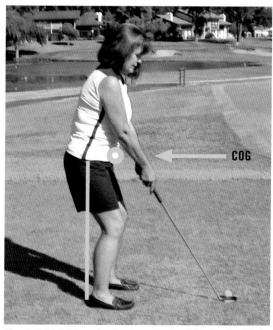

Fig. 5.9 Weight on the heels pulls the COG back with it.

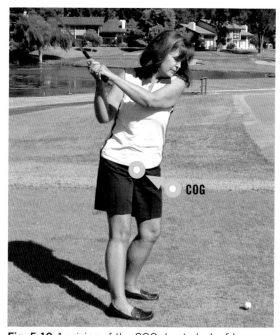

Fig. 5.10 A raising of the COG due to lack of lower-body stability

ity in the muscle chains of the body. The golf swing is really a lower-body game, yet most teachers only teach the upper-body movements.

When I was a teenager, I used to go down to UCLA and watch legendary coach John Wooden conduct his practices. Coach Wooden would have Lew Alcindor (later called Kareem Abdul-Jabbar) and his entire team perform footwork drills for the first part of practice. Even though golf doesn't require the jumping and running of basketball, it requires balance and stability to make a consistent golf swing. The drills that I prescribe for my students help promote this balance and stability. Without these two elements at the foundation of the golf swing, a golfer has little chance to improve, and all of the golf instruction that person receives will normally have minimal effect.

KINEMATIC SEQUENCING

Over the past several years, much fascinating research on the timing and sequencing of the movement of the body parts has been done with 3-D motion-capture systems. I believe that 3-D motion capture will be the teaching methodology of the future and will eventually replace 2-D video cameras, just as 2-D video cameras replaced giving lessons with the naked eye. Among other things, 3-D technology measures the timing and sequencing of the body parts throughout the swing; 2-D cameras simply can't measure these undetectable things. I call 3-D technology the "golf swing lie detector test" because everything you need to know is revealed. This technology has also shown that virtually all sports that involve hitting or

throwing an object have nearly the same kinematic sequencing on the forward motion of the activity.

This is what must happen in an effective golf swing, starting with the downswing: First, the hips begin to unwind and lead the way (as we've described in Chapters 3 and 4). The hips actually begin to shift and rotate before the club reaches the top of the backswing (this is very noticeable in a baseball pitcher's motion). While the hips are unwinding and the club is still going back, an increased stretch occurs between the upper- and lower-body parts. The "X factor stretch," as renowned golf instructor Jim McLean calls it, is increased. So, if at the top of the swing the hips have turned 45 degrees, and the shoulders 90 degrees, we have a 2:1 X factor. However, because the hips unwind first (a millisecond before the upper trunk unwinds and the club starts down), there is an actual increase in the X factor. In the case of a 45 degree: 90 degree hip and shoulder ratio, the unwinding of the hips can actually make it a 40 degree: 90 degree ratio. Some power hitters can actually increase it more. Nearly all great players have good kinematic sequencing, and very few (if any) bad players have good sequencing.

In proper sequencing, the hips lead the way, followed by the upper trunk, then the arms, and then the club (Fig. 5.11). When the forces of the unwinding of the hips shift over onto the left foot, they then come to an abrupt halt, which catapults the upper trunk, arms, and club, accelerating them through the shot. The peaking of these segments determines the efficiency of the swing. In kinematic-sequencing graphs, the lines peak above and slightly

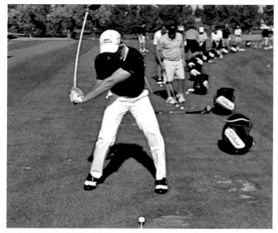

Fig. 5.11 Notice the explosive hip action of 2008 and 2009 RE/MAX World Long Drive champion Jamie Sadlowski.

forward of one another. To picture this, imagine a discus or javelin thrower hurling his body around and finally planting his front leg right before the throw. An instant after the planting of the foot, a shock wave is sent up the left leg, which forces the hip to clear, which forces the upper trunk to clear, which then allows the arm to swing through, hurling the object. Nearly all sports that involve throwing or hitting something have virtually the same kinematic sequencing.

Another example of kinematic sequencing is the action of cracking a whip. To get a good snap, a lion tamer cocks his wrist back, then snaps it forward, and at the last moment pulls the wrist and forearm back. In other words, the moment he brakes the wrist and begins to pull it back, the snap occurs. Looking at the golf swings of Jim Furyk and Ernie Els with the naked eye, you can see almost nothing remotely similar between them. Their kinematic-sequencing graphs, however, are amazingly similar. We can now look at the sequencing of

the graphs of many different players, and without having seen the golfer, we can tell with 100 percent accuracy who the best ball strikers are! It's that revealing.

The overwhelming majority of high handicappers have poor kinematic sequencing, and in nearly all of them, the hips, upper body, arms, and club are always out of sequence. The overwhelming majority of high handicappers start the downswing with the upper body and arms. If golfers don't load their hips effectively on their backswings, their chances of starting down with the pelvis first and then achieving good sequencing are very remote.

This exciting research regarding kinematic sequencing has changed our perspective on what makes a good golf swing. If the body parts are moving in sync, you're going to have much better contact with the ball. And if the muscles are flexible and strong, the sequencing and movement will be harmonious. In summary, the action of the hips will usually tell the story.

FLEXIBILITY TESTS
AND WHAT THEY MEAN

THIS CHAPTER IS DESIGNED to help you determine how flexible you are, and how your flexibility (or lack of it) is influencing your golf swing mechanics and your posture. We will do this through a series of simple but revealing range-of-motion tests. After all the years that I've administered these tests, I'm still amazed by how accurately they explain why a golfer does what he does in his swing. When you understand why your failure to perform a certain test effectively is directly related to your golf swing faults, you'll then be on your way to permanent improvement in both your body and your golf swing. I've come to call this the "magic moment," because when people begin to understand how the limitations in their bodies affect their golf swings (and they finally know what to do about it),

they begin to develop a great deal of enthusiasm and renewed hope in improving their golf swings.

For example, when a person fails in the hamstring test (the runner's stretch, S3, page 150), we normally see a straightening of the right leg, or an under position with their hips in the setup. I encourage you to be diligent in taking the tests because they will explain what's going on in your body and in your golf swing much more than you'd think. This will help you better understand the role that flexibility plays in the golf swing and, especially, in your golf swing. After helping you diagnose your golf swing characteristics, I will suggest some drills and specific flexibility stretches that will allow you to produce a freer and more functional golf swing. First, though, the tests.

TEST 1: **LAT TEST, PART 1**

Let's start with the lat test, which also tests the obliques and the pecs. This two-part test will reveal if you have any restriction in your upper torso and shoulders. The lat muscles (along the back and sides of the torso) as well as the obliques and pecs play an important role in the golf swing, and they are crucial in creating trunk rotation and extension for your arms. The lat muscles also stabilize the shoulders, so finding any limitations in their function is a big help in understanding and taking the necessary steps in improving your body and your golf swing. Common symptoms of tight lats and obliques are the collapsing of the arms on the backswing and forward swing (the chicken wing), as well as restrictions in making an efficient shoulder coil. So often people attempt to cure arm and chicken wing problems by putting an elastic band on their elbow joint to keep their left arm straight. In reality, though, the arms are only a symptom of the problem.

The problem usually can be found in the tightness of both sides of the body as well as the pecs. If we see a golfer whose head is tilted forward and whose back is rounded, we know this person has an imbalance in the relationship between the pec muscles and the lat muscles, as well as the rhomboids, traps, and levators. In other words, the chest muscles have become shortened and tighter, which in turn pulls the chest and shoulders forward. Rounded shoulders invariably restrict the chest from expanding on the backswing, preventing a full shoulder turn. (A person with these imbalances almost always has tight and dominant hips as well, contributing to the chest and shoulders being pulled in, but more on that later.)

This test may look simple, but the truth is that most people, especially seniors, have a very hard time doing this. An inability to pass this test almost certainly reveals a restricted shoulder turn in the golf swing. The body will desperately try to compensate in other areas. Many Champions Tour players exhibit a hunched back from the millions of golf swings they have produced over a lifetime; tight quadriceps and hips from walking thousands of fairway miles, standing on their feet for countless hours on the driving range and putting green, and the constant sitting down on airplanes and at dinner tables have also contributed to this condition; plus the swinging of their arms has helped strengthen the anterior muscles of their hips and shoulders.

STEP 1 Stand about 1½ feet away from a wall with your knees bent. Press your lower back, shoulders, and head against the wall, arms paral-

Fig. 6.1 Starting position **Fig. 6.2** Ending position

lel to the floor *(Fig. 6.1)*. If you can't get your head back to the wall comfortably, or if you do and your jawline is not parallel to the floor, you're being restricted by tight lats and pecs. As a result, your shoulder turn will be compromised.

STEP 2 Slowly raise your arms as high as you can (don't cheat, keep them straight). Do not let your lower back arch off the wall *(Fig 6.2)*.

RESULTS If your straight arms can easily go up and touch the wall and your back doesn't come off the wall, you have passed the test and most likely have a functional shoulder turn, one that properly coils and produces a lot of power into the shot. If you can't keep your arms straight and get your hands to touch the wall, and/or if your lower back begins to come off the wall (which is a compensation), you have restriction in your lats and thoracic/chest area.

TEST 1: **LAT TEST, PART 2**

STEP 1 Stand in the same position with your feet approximately 1 foot off the wall and your lower back and head against the wall. Check to see if your jawline is level or if your head isn't touching the wall. Now, place your arms flush against the wall in an eight o'clock and four o'clock position, with the backs of your hands against the wall *(Fig. 6.3)*.

STEP 2 Making sure your arms are ramrod straight, begin sliding your hands and arms up the wall as high as they'll go *(Fig. 6.4)*. Eventually, they're going to begin to bend and/or come off the wall.

RESULTS For functional lats, obliques, and pecs, you should be able to get your arms (while straight) at least to the 10 o'clock and two o'clock position. (Most people just get past nine

Fig. 6.3 Starting position

Fig. 6.4 Ending position

Fig. 6.5 Having the arms bent at this position indicates a failed test.

Fig. 6.6 Starting position

Fig. 6.7 Pike up, straighten your legs, and push your heels to the floor.

o'clock and three o'clock.) It's common for people to cheat by bending their arms as they slide up the wall. Make sure that you're diligent in maintaining perfect form during the tests. If you don't give yourself a true test, then you won't get a true assessment.

TEST 2: **LOWER HAMSTRING AND CALF TEST**

The downward dog test will help determine your calf and lower hamstring function. Without stable calves, there will be little chance of having a stable lower body in the golf swing. The calves are actually at the bottom of the posterior muscle chain, which runs from your heel up to your neck. Whenever I see a tight calf

muscle, I normally see a tight back. As strange as it may sound, the first step in straightening out a person's rounded shoulders is to start by loosening up the calves and hamstrings.

STEP 1 Remove your shoes and socks. Start on the floor on all fours with your hands directly underneath your shoulder joints and your knees directly underneath your hip joints *(Fig. 6.6)*.

STEP 2 Gently pike up by straightening your legs and pushing your heels to the floor. Keep your knees tight and raise your tailbone as high as you can *(Fig. 6.7)*.

RESULTS If you can get your heels to touch or get within $\frac{1}{2}$ inch of the floor, you have functional calves and good stability throughout your swing. If you can only get your heels to within 1 inch to $1\frac{1}{2}$ inches of the floor, then

Fig. 6.8 Severely restricted calves

Fig. 6.9 Starting position

your calves need some work. If your calves are 2 inches or higher from the floor *(Fig. 6.8)*, you have very tight calves and are severely restricted in your attempt to have a stable lower body in your golf swing. Tight calves work in unison with the hamstrings. If you have tight calves, you probably will have tight hamstrings (not to mention a tight back). In the next test, you will see just how these muscles affect your golf swing mechanics.

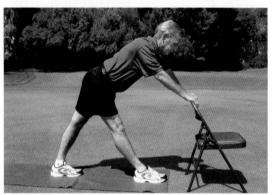

Fig. 6.10 Keep the legs straight and flatten the foot before starting down the chair.

TEST 3: **HAMSTRING TEST**

The hamstrings are connected to the pelvis and are a major influence in stabilizing the pelvis, as well as contributing to its rotation. Tight hamstrings prevent the pelvis from functioning properly throughout the swing. You will need a chair for this test.

STEP 1 From a kneeling position, start by putting your hands on the top of a chair. Place your right foot forward and bring your left knee flush against the back of your right heel *(Fig. 6.9)*.

STEP 2 Slowly stand up and straighten both legs and flatten the left foot *(Fig. 6.10)*.

Fig. 6.11 Ending position

STEP 3 Keeping both knees locked at all times, slowly walk your hands down the sides of the chair and see how close to the floor you can get without bending your knees *(Fig. 6.11)*. You will feel some pulling on the back side of your front knee in particular, but don't bend your knees. Keep them locked at all times. Most people cheat by bending the front knee in order to get their fingertips closer to the floor. Keeping your knees locked at all times is crucial in determining your hamstring function.

RESULTS If you can get your fingertips to touch or get within 1 to 2 inches of the floor, your hamstrings are functional and you don't have to worry about lower-body stability in your golf swing.

If you can only get your fingers and hands within 12 to 18 inches of the floor, you have very tight hamstrings. If you can't get your hands and fingertips to within 2 feet of the floor, you have severely dysfunctional hamstrings and definitely have some problems stabilizing your lower body in your swing, not to mention you'll be prone to back problems. An unstable lower body will certainly produce excessive and compensatory movements in your upper body during the swing. The best way to cure upper-body swing faults is to stabilize your lower body.

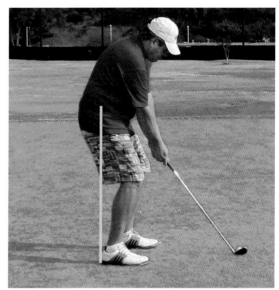

Fig. 6.12 Tight hamstrings will pull the golfer's hips backward, flattening the pelvis and putting the weight on the heels.

than it may appear *(Fig. 6.12)*. The hamstring muscles and the glutes must lengthen to accommodate this tilt, as the hip flexors then contract. In fact, there is a very high percentage of people who simply can't get into a proper address position due to dysfunctions of their hamstrings and glutes. Many simply tuck their hips under, and when told to get their butts up, they straighten their legs and lean too far forward.

If the hamstrings and glutes are tight, they won't allow the golfer to properly bend the hips forward because of the tightness of these muscles. The golfer will tend to sink backward on the heels, which will also raise the hands and arms at address. From this position, the golfer is doomed even before swinging the club because the muscles have little or no chance to stabilize the body, thus keeping the golfer out of balance.

COMMON SWING FAULTS CAUSED BY TIGHT HAMSTRINGS
Flattening of the Pelvis in the Address Position

When a golfer sets up in an address position, the pelvis must be tilted forward toward the ground. Tour players tilt their hips on average anywhere from 7 to 28 degrees. This seemingly simple move is very deceiving and much more difficult

Straightening of the Legs

As the upper-body weight shifts onto the right (or dominant) foot and leg, the front quadriceps and hip flexors begin to contract. This forces the hamstrings to expand. However, a tight hamstring (or a weak quadriceps) will not accept the forces being placed on it and the leg will usually straighten *(Fig. 6.13)*. Once the leg straightens, the hip becomes elevated, producing a chain reaction where virtually every part of the body becomes out of sequence. Golf swing mechanics are affected as well, usually resulting in a laying off of the club, followed by a lifting of the club, then an over-the-top move.

Fig. 6.13 Straightening of the legs is usually due to tight hamstrings and hips.

A straightening of the right (or dominant) leg usually results in the weight shifting back onto the heels. This move also takes the contraction out of the legs and throws the body out of balance because the center of gravity has been moved rearward. Remember, for every centimeter the center of gravity shifts, the clubhead can move up to 14 inches out of its proper relationship, or orbit, with the center. With the contraction now taken out of the lower body, the resistance and dynamic tension of the upper body is lost, the shoulder coil becomes slackened, and the hands and arms usually begin flailing away, trying to find their way back home—back to the ball, just like the tightrope walker's pole when he loses his balance on the high wire.

Flattening of the Shoulders

Because big muscles control little muscles, when the right leg begins to straighten, the direction of the forces is pulled inside and the shaft is sucked along with it. The club will then "lay off" and swing on a flatter swing plane. Again, much like the tightrope walker, the body, always seeking balance, will recognize this and begin to lift the club (the pole) in an effort to regain balance. The club then begins its journey outside and over the top, a move that all golfers try to avoid.

The shoulders in a functional golf swing should maintain their 90-degree relationship with the spine angle that was established in the address position. In other words, at the top of the swing, the clavicles should be pointing down and perpendicular to the spine, which is usually set at a 35- to 45-degree angle.

Another way to picture this is the shoulders at the top of the backswing should be parallel

Fig. 6.14 Arnold Palmer shows perfect tilt and turn of his shoulders.

Fig. 6.15 A typical laying off and flattening of the shoulders

to the shaft angle established at address *(Fig. 6.14)*. However, when the right leg straightens due to tight hamstrings, the pelvis will usually over-rotate, which in turn affects the spine and shoulders. The shoulders are now drawn into the act and they too begin to flatten *(Fig. 6.15)*, coming out of the spine angle created at address. Since the shoulders control the arms, the arms lose control, and in turn, the wrists will not hinge in the proper sequence.

Because the hamstrings also have a major influence on the pelvis, this tightening usually restricts the freedom of the hips in not only the backswing but also the forward swing. Without pelvic rotation, the golfer cannot effectively shift his weight with the lower body and therefore will not be able to maximize clubhead speed.

This usually results in "no cheeks" at impact. Because the hamstrings are tight, this

results in an early straightening of the left leg as the golfer swings into the shot (just the reverse of the backswing). It is okay for the left leg to straighten, but it has to come after the weight has already shifted to the left foot. A premature straightening of the left leg forces the hips and shoulders to brake too soon, which usually produces an out-to-in swing path coming into the ball. As a result, the ball will start out to the left.

Lack of Arm Extension

Because tight hamstrings tend to straighten the legs and produce a premature braking action, this also causes the hips to jam. Once the hips jam and stop rotating, the centrifugal force generated by the body is interrupted and the arms lose their extension, resulting in the infamous chicken wing finish.

This dreaded position is the result of the collision between the body and the arms. The straightening of the leg is often the reason for the premature uncocking of the wrists.

So, tight calves and hamstrings play a big role in every action in the upper body and arms. Even a slight increase in the range of motion in the calves and hamstrings makes a huge difference in producing a functional golf swing.

TEST 4: **HIP FLEXOR TEST (THE THOMAS TEST)**

This test will tell a lot about the functioning of your hips. How the hips function in the golf swing (and in every sport for that matter) is paramount. Even the slightest movement of the hips will affect every joint in the body. If you are overweight, this test won't be accurate; proceed to the alternate test that follows.

STEP 1 Sit on the edge of a massage table (or the top of a stairwell, a countertop, or table). Make sure that the middle of your thighs are on the edge of the table.

STEP 2 From the sitting position, roll onto your back while simultaneously taking hold of each knee with your hands just below the kneecaps. Roll all the way back and allow your head to rest on the table.

STEP 3 With your head on the table, pull your knees back as far as you can toward your shoulders *(Fig. 6.16)*.

STEP 4 Take your right hand off your right knee and put it on your left knee, assisting the left hand. Using both hands, keep pulling your left knee even more, so that it draws even closer

to your left shoulder *(Fig. 6.17)*. Slowly relax your right leg and let it come back down toward the table. Don't force your right leg down; let it come down very s-l-o-w-l-y.

RESULTS If your right hip is functional, your entire right leg will settle directly onto the table *(Fig. 6.18)*. This is rare, however. If your leg doesn't return flat on the table but instead produces a gap between the leg and the table *(Fig. 6.19)*, you definitely have a tight right hip. Be

Fig. 6.16 Knees back toward shoulders as far as possible

Fig. 6.17 Pull the left knee toward the left shoulder and slowly lower the right leg down toward the table.

Fig. 6.18 Functional hip

Fig. 6.19 Tight hip

sure to repeat on the other side and compare. Excess baby fat around your midsection won't allow an accurate test, so if that's the case, take the alternate test that follows.

ALTERNATE HIP FLEXOR TEST

Follow step 1 of the hip flexor test. Roll back on the table and pull back your left knee with your left hand. Place your right hand under the small of your back *(Fig. 6.20)*. When you pull your left knee back, check to see if your right leg rises off the table. If it does, you have a tight right hip. If it severely comes off the table, you have a very tight right hip. Also, check to see if the right calf (which was hanging off the table) has shifted. If it has elevated upward, it is also an indication that you have an overly tight right quadriceps (quad). If this is the case, you definitely have tight quads and hip flexors. Tight hips hinder every aspect of your golf swing. Your hips will have a difficult time blending the proper amount of rotation and stability throughout your swing, and you will often "compensate for compensations."

Fig. 6.20 Alternate test. Note how the right thigh has lifted off the table and that the right lower leg is not pointing straight down, indicating a tight hip and quad.

EFFECTS ON THE GOLF SWING A tight dominant hip is the number one problem in golf, for it affects everything. People with overdeveloped quads, such as bicyclists, marathon runners, skiers, and bodybuilders, tend to lose their rotational capacity due to the overdevelopment of their quads and hips. Overstrengthening a muscle shortens it. When it is shortened, it doesn't move efficiently. This in turn reduces a muscle's rotational capacity.

Let's look at golfers with this condition. When they begin to shift their upper-body weight in the backswing, the tight hips usually don't allow them to achieve a natural rotation. As a result, the hips tend to slide out to the right. This move is usually catastrophic and leads to many other faults, such as moving the weight to the outside of the right foot, forcing the upper body into a reverse mode, flattening the shoulders, and producing a flying right elbow. Why the elbow? Remember the sequence of the body: legs control hips, hips control shoulders, shoulders control arms, and arms control hands. If the hips are tight, the odds are that the chest will be tight, and if the chest is tight, it won't expand, forcing the arms to collapse.

In the backswing, when the hips begin to turn, the shoulders begin to turn. They turn on the axis of the spine, which is tilted forward about 35 to 45 degrees. The left shoulder will tilt down approximately 6 to 8 inches, and the right shoulder will rise up about the same amount. What happens when the right shoulder rises? The right arm has no choice but to fold, which in turn folds the wrists, which cocks the club. When the right hip slides, this stops the proper rotation of the hips. It also impedes the rotation of the shoulders, which in turn prevents the right arm from folding. In an attempt to gain freedom, the right arm then begins to fly and lift up and outward from its intended plane.

One of the biggest swing faults is the blocking of the hips at impact—no two-cheek position. The proper rotation of the hips on the forward swing is just not there. A sliding hip usually creates a reverse tilt of the upper body, so the upper body wants to get back in position by moving first on the downswing. The upper body and especially the left shoulder must stay behind the left leg at all times until the majority of the weight shifts onto the left foot. The lower body must initiate the downswing, followed by the trunk, arms, hands, and clubhead.

Tight hips are responsible for other swing faults, namely too much hip turn and, at times, too much shoulder turn. Too much hip and shoulder turn on the backswing will usually lead to not enough hip and shoulder turn on the forward swing. In other words, we want to create a maximum amount of separation or torque in the midsection of our body. This is the result of a stable lower body and a fully coiled upper body.

If a person's hips are too tight, there will usually not be adequate torque (X factor). Because the body knows it can't create separation between the lower trunk and the upper trunk, the hips and shoulders will overturn. A 45-degree hip turn and a 90-degree shoulder turn will produce a 2:1 ratio. If a golfer turns his hips 70 degrees and his shoulders 120 degrees, they have decreased the amount of torque and coil they are trying to achieve.

Invariably, an overturn of both the hips and shoulders results in a straightening of the right leg. By now, we all know what that produces.

TEST 5: **SHOULDER TURN TEST**

Everybody in golf wants a bigger shoulder turn, and for good reason. Coiling the shoulders properly against the resistance of the lower body pays huge dividends. It produces power and consistency, which mean longer and straighter drives and more greens in regulation. Getting all that body mass behind the ball and then releasing it is imperative in the golf swing. The problem, however, is that very few people are capable of making the big turn that they see the Tour players make so effortlessly. The average golfer is incapable of making a true 90-degree shoulder turn. As a result, he usually gets in a world of trouble when trying to do so. This test shows you just how much of a turn you can make.

STEP 1 Start by sitting down on the floor with your legs extended. Sitting upright, bring your right foot over your left leg, just outside the knee. If you can't get your right foot up as high, or higher, than your knee, it's not a big deal, just place it farther down your leg, closer to your left foot. Just make sure you keep your foot flat on the floor.

STEP 2 Place your right hand directly behind you so that your fingers are pointing directly away from you, ideally in the midline of your body. Keep your left arm straight and place it across your chest so that it is pressing onto your right thigh. Turn your head as far behind you

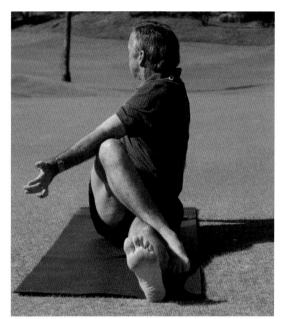

Fig. 6.21 Shoulders in line with extended left leg indicating functional upper-torso turn

Fig. 6.22 Example of a failed shoulder turn test: The student is unable to get her shoulders in line with her extended leg.

as you can, theoretically looking over your right shoulder *(Fig. 6.21)*.

RESULTS Now check out the position of your shoulders. If they are not in line with your extended left leg, you lack the flexibility necessary to make a true 90-degree shoulder turn *(Fig. 6.22)*. In fact, looking at the angle of your shoulders in relation to your extended left leg will almost invariably give you the number of degrees that you can turn your shoulders. In other words, if your shoulders are approximately 75 degrees in line with your leg, you can probably make a 75-degree shoulder turn (without cheating).

What do I mean by cheating? The following test will give you a clear understanding of the relationship between the shoulders and hips and how they synchronize with each other.

ALTERNATE SHOULDER TURN TEST

STEP 1 You will need a block or other prop for this test. Lie on the floor in a fetal position with your thighs angled 90 degrees from your torso and your lower legs angled 90 degrees from your thighs *(Fig. 6.23)*. Place your arms directly out in front of you with your hands in prayer.

STEP 2 Keeping your knees together (and without letting your top knee slide off) and pressed against the block, swing your top hand and arm all the way back over to the floor. Let your head come back so that you're looking straight up at the ceiling *(Fig. 6.24)*. *(Again, don't let the top knee leave its original position.)* Most people can't get their top arm on the floor *(Fig. 6.25)*. How far your arm is off the floor will tell you just how far you can turn your shoulders.

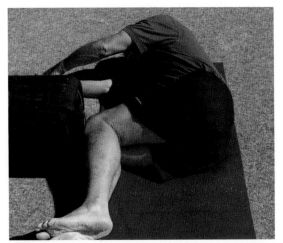

Fig. 6.23 Lower legs angled 90 degrees from thighs and thighs angled 90 degrees from torso

Fig. 6.24 Top hand and arm swung back with head turned to face up

Fig. 6.25 Failed test

If you can't get your arm and shoulder on the floor, what's the only way that you can? Let go of your legs and you'll see.

As you release your top knee and leg, you'll notice that your arm and shoulder hit the floor. Is this a true shoulder turn? Of course not. By letting go of your leg, you've lost all the torque and coil that you've stored up. In other words, you've lost your X factor. This is a clear example of what the body does in the golf swing when it is physically unable to perform a movement. Other parts of the body help out and compensate. The body then begins to compensate for compensations, and the entire kinetic chain of dominoes becomes chaos.

TEST 6: **SITTING FLOOR TEST**

I love this stretch, although most people hate it, including Arnold Palmer (at least he used to). When I put Mr. Palmer into this stretch the first day I worked with him, I thought it might be the end of our new relationship. He wasn't happy sitting against that wall down at Bay Hill. Many of you won't be happy either (at first).

The good news is that by diligently practicing this and the rest of the stretches in my program (see Chapter 11), you will come to look forward to this pose—just like Arnold Palmer does. More good news: The easier this pose gets, the better your golf swing will function, guaranteed! This not only stretches out the muscles in the lower body (specifically, calves, hamstrings, and glutes), it also coordinates all of the muscles along the entire posterior muscle chain. In other words, it stretches all the muscles up the back as well. Believe it or not, your body wants to be in this position and, in time, will do it easily.

STEP 1 Sit as close to a wall as you possibly can, ideally with your tailbone touching the wall. Keep your legs straight with your knees pressed together and pressing into the floor. If your knees don't quite make it, don't worry about it. Arch your feet straight back toward you *(Fig. 6.26)*.

STEP 2 Do a shoulder shrug using your upper body, and try to get your shoulder blades flush against the wall. Place the back of your head against the wall with your chin down toward your sternum. Your jaw should be parallel to the floor. This position is your goal. If you can't get into it, that's okay for now. If you can't keep your legs straight on the floor, your knees together, or your chin down and your shoulders back, don't force it. Just be aware of where your body is.

Fig. 6.26 Starting position

Fig. 6.27 Failed test

RESULTS If you can't keep your legs down or in a straight line, you have hamstring and lower-body dysfunction. If you can't keep your back against the wall while your jawline is level, you have tightness in your upper chest and shoulders *(Fig. 6.27)*. As far as your golf swing goes, since your chest is too tight and won't expand, you will have a hard time getting your back to the target. How well you perform this test will demonstrate how well your upper trunk and your lower torso work with one another. If you can't do this test very well, you won't be able to maintain lower-body stability in your swing. When you are able to do the sitting wall test comfortably, you will be amazed at how this will positively affect your golf swing. Because all the muscle chains will be in sync, you will be able to maintain both stability and your spine angle. This pose will probably test you, but it will also tell you a lot about where you are (or aren't) and where you need to go.

SUMMARY

Although I've isolated these tests and pointed out how your performance in them influences your golf swing mechanics, the body has a magnificent way of compensating for compensations. In other words, you may fail in some of the tests and not have the swing faults that have been described here. This means that some muscles in other parts of the body have picked up the slack and taken over for your dysfunctional muscles.

The greater your range of motion and muscle function, the more efficient your movement. This smooth-working kinetic chain will produce a freer, more powerful golf swing.

CHAPTER 7

FLEXIBLE SOLUTIONS TO INFLEXIBLE SWING FAULTS

AS FAR AS I KNOW, nobody in history has achieved a perfect golf swing. Everyone has some unorthodox characteristic in their swing that is unique to them, whether it's Jack Nicklaus's flying right elbow, Tiger Woods's dip into the ball, or Sam Snead's slight inside-and-over move. Even Ernie Els's magnificent swing sometimes has a little hitch at the top of his backswing. Everybody has something in their swing that they fight for a lifetime.

The big question is: Are these faults just habits, or are they symptoms of that individual's anatomical function or dysfunction? I've learned that, most of the time, it is the latter. In other words, your body is your golf swing, and to cure these faults one must usually start with changing one's body and anatomical function.

Golfers have taken millions of lessons,

which have included endless theories and philosophies on how to fix and cure swing faults. Golfers are constantly thinking of how this little adjustment or that new move will magically cure their faults and create a more effective swing. This has gone on for hundreds of years and probably will go on for eternity. Very seldom do quick fixes really fix a golf swing for an extended period. Most players will try another tip as soon as the current one stops working. There really is no answer. Or is there?

The very premise of this book is to help people realize that for hundreds of years there has been a myth in the game of golf: The myth is that just by working on golf swing mechanics or by taking lessons a golfer will be able to fix or correct swing faults. But it doesn't always work that way.

The notion that practice makes perfect, or even that perfect practice makes perfect, is not necessarily true, especially as golfers reach senior status. Most seniors should focus more on improving their flexibility and less on perfecting their golf swings. Again, your body is your golf swing.

It is widely believed that hard work, dedication, and persistence are the keys to great golf, yet most golfers do not automatically improve simply by taking lessons or working diligently on their swings. Why is it so hard for most people to correct the faults or tendencies in their golf swings?

Yes, golfers sometimes fall into habits that are fixed by rudimentary instruction. However, in most cases, in order to make an effective change in a person's swing, the functioning of that person's body has to be changed.

As an example, an elderly golfer (72 to 75 years old) came to see me for a golf lesson. Before we got started, I asked him about his goals and expectations from this lesson. (There are always two stock answers: (1) to be more consistent, and (2) to hit the ball farther, or both.) This gentleman replied that his main goal was to gain more distance. I asked him if he expected to hit the ball as far as Tiger Woods when the lesson was over. As I expected, he looked at me quizzically and replied, "Are you some sort of comedian? Of course not. I could never hit the ball as far as Tiger Woods." I said, "Tell me exactly why you don't think you ever could." The man replied, "Because he's nearly three times younger than I am!" I then responded, "What exactly does being younger have to do with it?" I could see the man's frustration rising, but he did give me the right answer. He simply said, "Hell, he's much

stronger than me, he's much more flexible than me, he has more vitality, and his nerves are better than mine!"

This was exactly what I was trying to get him to say. I then said, "Oh, so if that's the case, wouldn't you agree that if we got you stronger, more flexible, with more energy and vitality, you'd probably gain the distance that you're looking for?" With a newfound enlightenment, the man looked at me and said, "Of course, but at my age, is it even possible to regain strength and flexibility?" "Absolutely," I said. I told him he could get it back, but not by just taking a golf lesson. By doing the proper stretches, in the correct way, and by following a regular fitness program, he definitely could regain much of the strength and flexibility he had lost. Furthermore, an increased range of motion, along with more power generated from his body, would automatically result in more clubhead speed and more power in his shots.

To most golfers this is obvious. The truth is that most people fail to look at their golf swings from this perspective and fail to recognize that their body is indeed their swing. Instead, they usually have the misconception that finding the right swing tip will provide the ultimate answer to their golf swing troubles. Always remember that just working on the new Tour move isn't going to grow a new hip flexor or hamstring! To repeat, your swing faults will more than likely remain, especially if you're getting older, unless you change your anatomical function and especially your range of motion. So many older people tell me, "I'm too old to exercise and do all that stuff." To them I say, "You're too old not to."

In this chapter we're going to take a look at several of golf's most common swing faults and explain how these particular faults are usually symptoms of a lack of flexibility and strength in certain muscle groups of the body. Each swing fault will have a menu of stretches, exercises, and swing drills that will help remove that fault once and for all. By combining the stretches (in Chapter 11) and the drills (in Chapter 8), you should be able to make some permanent changes in your body. Subsequently, you should be able to make a freer and more powerful golf swing.

Do these exercises for 7 to 10 days, and then the normal stretching protocols in Chapter 10, or simply combine them with your normal daily stretching program.

FAULT NO. 1: **POOR ADDRESS AND TAKEAWAY PROBLEMS**

A good golf swing must begin in balance. If a golfer is out of balance in the setup, virtually everything that happens from that point on will be a compensation, and often, compensations for compensations will follow. Much like the domino effect, how the first domino falls will influence all of the other dominoes in the chain.

I've learned through a lifetime of golf that getting into a balanced address position is often taken for granted by not only students but even some instructors. People who have tight quads, hips, and hamstrings not only have a difficult time assuming the address position, in many cases they are physically unable to do it correctly. I've also learned that there have been many different definitions of balance, but the truth is that physiologically there are only a few key points. They are as follows:

1. The weight must be 50-50 on each foot with the majority of the weight being on the balls of the feet just under the shoelaces.

2. The hip joints must align directly on top of the ankle joints.

We also like to see the knees over the shoelaces and the shoulder joints just outside the toes. From there, the arms will be allowed to hang comfortably downward. If these two factors aren't met, the golfer is, pure and simple, out of balance.

For many centuries, most golf instruction taught us to sit back on the heels, and the majority of golfers do tend to sit back on their heels, which in turn rounds their shoulders. But if a golfer keeps the weight on his heels, it is impossible for him to shift his weight effectively throughout the swing. When the weight

Fig. 7.1 Weight on heels. Note how the hip joint is outside the ankle.

is on the heels *(Fig. 7.1)*, the back will tend to round, which will influence a flat shoulder plane, coupled with a lifting of the arms as the golfer goes into his backswing.

Most poor takeaway problems come from a poor address position, which, as mentioned above, is usually caused by tight quads, hamstrings, and hips, and also by restrictions in the upper torso. We want the weight to move smoothly and effortlessly into the right foot and leg so as to load the hip. The best way to do this is to have the weight distributed evenly before the initial takeaway.

If, however, a golfer begins to shift into the right foot, and the aforementioned muscles are tight or weak, the lower-body muscles will not accept the forces placed upon them and will

tend to bail out, resulting in a straightening of the leg and an elevation of the hip *(Fig. 7.2)*. As the leg straightens, the shoulders also follow suit and begin to flatten, which will usually pull the shaft to the inside. Now too inside, and the club feeling heavy, the golfer will instinctively lift the shaft up and begin the path to the infamous over-the-top move. Imagine the tightrope walker on the high wire. For every centimeter he moves out of balance, he will counter with the balance pole in an effort to regain balance and equilibrium. The body and the shaft of the golf club react in precisely the same way.

The best way to get set up properly and take the club away smoothly is to have a balanced set of muscles throughout your torso. After all, how can you take a person with poor posture and suddenly expect him to achieve good posture in the setup?

The most common golf swing faults in the takeaway that I see are:

1. Straightening of the right leg
2. Improper loading of the hips (either overturning or underturning)
3. Yanking the club to the inside
4. Flattening the shoulders
5. Reversing
6. Breaking the wrists too early often leads to overturning and/or sliding the hips

The following drills and stretches will help you achieve a solid address position and help you make a proper takeaway.

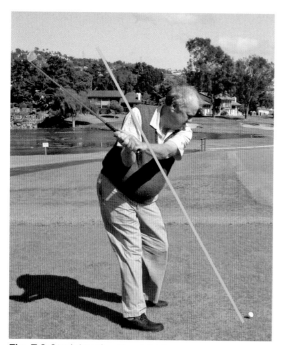

Fig. 7.2 Straightening the right leg

Golf Swing Drills

1. Close-the-eyes balance drill (D1, page 91)

2. Foam-roller drill (D3, page 94)

3. Push-away drill (D5, page 99)

4. Baseball drill (D8, page 102)

Stretches

1. Counter (S22, page 165)

2. Downward dog (S1, page 149)

3. Runner's stretch (S3, page 150)

(continued)

Stretches—cont.

4. Extended lateral
(S27, page 168)

5. Spread-foot forward bend
(S2, page 150)

6. Psoas stretch
(S14, page 158)

7. Hip-thigh extension
(S18, page 161)

8. Lateral ball roll
(S41, page 183)

9. Wall squat (S49, page 190)

FAULT NO. 2: **HIP SLIDING (AND NO CHEEKS)**

Another dangerous fault is the sliding of the hips, especially on the backswing. This swing fault is normally a result of tight hip flexors and tight quads and is especially common with bicyclists, marathoners, skiers, and bodybuilders. These athletes tend to overtrain and overdevelop their legs and hips in these types of activities. When a muscle gets overstrengthened, it tends to shorten and tighten. When a muscle gets shortened, it simply won't move as well. From my perspective, a muscle that doesn't move is a weak muscle. We want a muscle that moves easily and fluidly throughout its entire motion.

Tight quads and hip flexors make it difficult for the hip muscles to rotate properly. As a

Fig. 7.3 Classic hip slide

upper body starts down before the lower body, there is certainly trouble ahead. This is the most common fault among higher handi-cappers, as seen in the kinematic-sequencing graphs. Starting down with the upper body first is probably the most common fault in golf, and again, it is nearly always a symptom of the lower body not being able to stabilize and allow the twisting and turning of the upper body against it.

When the upper body starts down first, the club usually comes crashing down on a path that is over the shoulder and down into the ball at a steep angle—that is, over the top.

When the lower body initiates the down-ward swing, the arms and club drop down at a shallow angle, coming in from behind the ball, not on top of it. The answer to this swing fault is to simply stretch and relax the legs and hips (and often to strengthen the glutes), which allows the lower body to stabilize and create a dynamic stretch between the upper and lower torsos. Use the following drill and stretches to regain proper hip rotation and function.

result, when the weight begins to shift into the hips, the muscles do not have the capacity to rotate properly, and they begin to slide out to the right.

When the hip begins sliding, this usually forces the upper spine to reverse, or point back to the target *(Fig. 7.3)*. The center of gravity now leans back toward the left and not behind the ball as we want. Because the upper body hasn't moved behind the lower body (and allowed the lower body to initiate the forward swing), the upper body takes over and begins its wild descent into the ball (what I call the "Leaning Tower of Pisa"). If the

Golf Swing Drill

1. Elbow-to-wall drill (D6, page 100)

Stretches

1. Standing drop-off (with gluteal contractions) (S12, page 156)

2. Active groin stretch (S13, page 157)

3. Supine leg chain (S7, page 153)

4. Psoas stretch (S14, page 158)

5. Internal and external hip rotators (S20, page 163)

6. Hip crossover (S19, page 162)

7. Pretzel (S31, page 172)

8. Solo sitting wall (S17, page 160)

9. Supine groin stretch (S54, page 193)

FAULT NO. 3: **RESTRICTED SHOULDER TURN AND RESTRICTED FOLLOW-THROUGH**

Everybody wants to make a bigger shoulder turn and understandably so. The problem is that if you don't have flexible hips or a flexible upper torso, it's not going to happen *(Fig. 7.4)*. However, by maintaining a solid brace with your lower body, you'll automatically create a bigger X factor. For the average player with restricted flexibility, a smaller hip turn on the backswing is preferable to a big hip and shoulder turn. One of my pet peeves is that some golf instruction advises tight seniors to turn out the right foot in order to make a bigger hip turn. Although this indeed will create a bigger hip turn, it usually unplugs the golfer and dissipates the crucial resistance between the lower body and upper body.

No question about it, good golf demands flexibility in the upper trunk, primarily in the obliques, lats, chest, and lumbar muscles. Trunk flexibility is probably more important in golf than in any other sport. Golfers with rounded shoulders have a problem because, among other things, rounded shoulders indicate an overdominance and tightness of the pec muscles, which are required to expand on the backswing. Rounded shoulders basically mean that the front muscles of the chest are too tight and the back muscles are too weak.

The upper spine rotates approximately 60 percent more on the backswing than the lower spine, so if a person's shoulders are too tight, they won't allow the upper spine to rotate to its maximum. This rounded-shoulder condition, called thoracic kyphosis, is commonly seen among seniors and even Champions Tour play-

ers, who evolve into this condition, and who also eventually end up with very tight hips. This evolution is caused by walking thousands of miles around golf courses, tilting forward in a golf stance (which puts the hips in flexion), hitting millions of golf balls, sitting down in airplanes, driving cars, and so forth. It's no wonder that we see this hunchbacked position in so many senior golfers.

Having a flexible upper trunk and back can make up for a lot of other physical faults in the golf swing, and it makes it much easier to get the arms and club behind the body in the proper sequence. The following drills and stretches will help to increase your shoulder coil.

Fig. 7.4 Restricted shoulder turn

Golf Swing Drills

1. Elbow-to-wall drill
(D6, page 100)

2. Set, turn, and place drill
(D7, page 101)

Stretches

1. Standing drop-off
(with gluteal contractions)
(S12, page 156)

2. Cats and dogs
(S23, page 165)

3. Downward dog
(S1, page 149)

4. Triangle
(S26, page 167)

5. Psoas stretch
(S14, page 158)

6. Oblique side flex
(S30, page 171)

7. Pretzel
(S31, page 172)

8. Pectorals stretch
(S36, page 177)

Restricted Follow-Through

A simple comparison of the finish of a Tour player versus that of a high handicapper usually tells the whole story. The overwhelming majority of Tour players finish completely on their left sides and, in most cases, with their chests aiming to the left of the target *(Fig. 7.5)*. The high handicapper seldom comes close to this full finish position, usually ending up with an abbreviated finish or incomplete follow-through *(Fig. 7.6)*.

Most golfers lack the necessary flexibility to finish all the way around, the same way they lack the flexibility to get into a perfect backswing position. The golf swing drills and stretches on the opposite page will help you accomplish a full finish.

FAULT NO. 4: **LOSS OF SPINE ANGLE**

Keeping one's spine angle is paramount for hitting solid and consistent shots. The reason it's so important is that when a golfer comes out of his spine angle *(Fig. 7.7)*, he is really altering the center of gravity and losing energy, plus he is taking his muscles out of contraction. However, I must make note that when a golfer stands tall in the address position and actually lowers himself as he starts down, energy is actually increased. This move has been seen in many of golf's greatest players, including Tiger Woods, Byron Nelson, and thousands of other players. In fact, I would say that the majority of great players go down into the shot. Conversely, you'll seldom ever see a great player

Fig. 7.5 David Duval completely "unwound"

Fig. 7.6 Abbreviated follow-through

rising up. But, coming up and out of one's spine angle is very common among high handicappers.

When a golfer rises up as he comes into the ball, the torque and force are lost and, as a result, the club is released too soon. This will almost invariably result in a hand flip through the ball.

Another negative of coming out of the spine angle is that it normally puts the weight back on the heels, consequently taking the brace and stability out of the lower body. There are a few players who "back out" of their spine angle going through the ball, but that happens only with the driver. Because the ball is teed up, a person can get away with it a little more with the driver than with an iron. Once again, having a very stable and flexible body (especially lower body) will nearly always ensure maintaining a level spine angle. Here are some drills and stretches to help maintain your spine angle.

Fig. 7.7 A loss of spine angle due to restricted muscles

Golf Swing Drills

1. Brush-the-grass drill (D15, page 111)

2. Flagstick drill (D20, page 115)

Stretches

1. Counter (S22, page 165)

2. Downward dog (S1, page 149)

3. Runner's stretch
(S3, page 150)

4. Extended lateral
(S27, page 168)

5. Spread-foot forward bend
(S2, page 150)

6. Psoas stretch (S14, page 158)

7. Hip-thigh extension
(S18, page 161)

8. Lateral ball roll
(S41, page 183)

9. Wall squat (S49, page 190)

FAULT NO. 5: **FLYING ELBOWS AND CHICKEN WINGS**

A flying right elbow (made famous by Jack Nicklaus, Freddie Couples, and others) isn't necessarily a bad thing *(Fig. 7.8)*. The elbow and arm function is dictated by an individual's scapulas (or shoulder blades), and the rhomboid muscles, in conjunction with lats and pecs, greatly influence the scapulas. In addition, people with thick chests normally have thick backs and therefore don't have a lot of range of motion in their shoulder blades. Remember that the shoulders control the arms and the arms control the hands. Thick chests also inhibit a golfer's arms from folding naturally and easily. With a lack of shoulder blade rotation, the arms tend to lift or stray away from the body.

Golfers whose backs and chests aren't as broad tend to keep their elbows closer to their sides. One of Nicklaus's concerns was that sometimes his right elbow would fly too much and cause him to lift up out of his backswing. When this occurred, his head would rise and his left heel would also come up too high off of the ground. Consequently, his left foot would come crashing down prematurely and he would be prone to hit a pull hook. (Obviously, this didn't happen too much.)

Chicken wings occur on the forward swing in much the same way as a flying elbow on the backswing, again due to muscle restrictions in the upper torso and, especially, the shoulders. What generally happens is the left side of the body doesn't shift and rotate out of the way, which causes the arms to crash into the blocked torso, forcing them to collapse. In other words,

Fig. 7.8 Freddie Couples is living proof that a flying right elbow isn't necessarily a bad thing.

the chicken wing is actually a result of the lack of rotation of the upper torso and shoulder joints. The fact is people with tight lats, obliques, and impinged shoulders are very prone to the dreaded chicken wing. People are forever putting towels and gloves under their left armpits, using straps, and trying many other remedies to stay connected. These aids may help some, but the best way to cure this problem is to go to the source and loosen up the main muscles that are creating the problem in the first place. These drills and stretches should help get to the root of the problem.

Golf Swing Drills

1. Connection drill (D19, page 114)

2. Right-arm-only drill (D12, page 107)

Stretches

1. Standing drop-off (with gluteal contractions) (S12, page 156)

2. Overhead extension (S35, page 176)

3. Downward dog (S1, page 149)

4. Psoas stretch (S14, page 158)

5. Russian ball twist (S34, page 175)

6. Lateral ball roll (S41, page 183)

7. Internal and external shoulder rotators (S42, page 184)

8. Why me (S39, page 181) and Breaststroke (S40, page 182)

FAULT NO. 6: **DOWNSWING PROBLEMS**

These are five common downswing faults:

1. Coming over the top *(Fig. 7.9)*
2. Lack of lower body stability
3. Getting stuck on the right side
4. Straightening the legs
5. Upper body starting down first

Without question, how we come into the ball is the most important aspect of the swing and truly is the make-or-break moment. We must initiate the downswing with the unwinding of the hips. In fact, there really is no top of the backswing because the hips actually begin unwinding a split second before the club reaches the top. This move actually increases the X factor on the backswing and is a common trait among power hitters.

As the hips are unwinding, the center of gravity moves forward as the weight shifts onto the left foot. The forces on the foot then create a shock wave that rushes back up the femur, causing the hips to clear. When the hips begin the process of starting down, the chain reaction begins: the upper trunk unwinds, the arms and club drop down between the right shoulder and the right hip, and finally the hands follow into impact. The result of this sequencing creates centrifugal force, which causes the wrists to lag behind the arms and body, storing up maximum power for the release yet to come. However, if this sequencing is out of order, there will be an interruption of the synchronization of these body parts. If the upper body starts down first (and not the lower), the hips usually will come to a crashing halt far too soon, creating a premature uncocking of the wrists and often the aforementioned chicken wing *(Fig. 7.10)*.

Here are some drills and stretches to create a maximum lower body move into the ball and help shift the weight and clear the hips.

Fig. 7.9 Over the top

Fig. 7.10 Getting stuck on the right side

Golf Swing Drills

1. Step-on-the-gas drill
(D13, page 109)

2. Right-arm-only drill
(D12, page 107)

3. Wall-press drill
(D16, page 112)

4. Baseball drill
(D8, page 102)

Stretches

1. Cats and dogs
(S23, page 165)

2. Cobra
(S25, page 166)

3. Downward dog
(S1, page 149)

4. Warrior II
(S15, page 159)

5. Triangle
(S26, page 167)

6. Extended lateral
(S27, page 168)

7. Pretzel in chair
(S31A, page 172)

8. Air bench
(S51, page 192)

As strange as this may sound, having tight pecs or a tight upper torso also will cause the chicken wing because of the chest's lack of capacity to expand and properly rotate on the backswing, which will not allow the push-pull sequence to occur. Again, the transition sequence from the top of the swing down is the make-or-break moment in the golf swing.

Straightening of the Legs

Like every other sport, golf is a lower-body game. Although the vast majority of golf instruction centers on upper-body swing mechanics and swing positions, the lower-body stability allows the upper body to do its thing. One such swing fault that is guaranteed to disrupt the stabilization of the golf swing is a premature straightening of the legs, especially the left leg, as the golfer transitions into the downswing *(Fig. 7.11)*. This locking-up causes a braking motion that disrupts the rhythm and forces as they flow into impact.

A lot of teachers advocate a straightening of the left leg at impact to generate more shock power through the shot. I have no problem with this, except that it is a highly skilled move that requires precise timing. The vast majority of amateur golfers simply can't perform this move with precision. Keeping the knees flexed through the shot is almost considered taboo by many of today's teachers, but guys like Byron Nelson, Ben Hogan *(Fig. 7.12)*, Jack Nicklaus, Tommy Bolt, George Knudson, Johnny Miller, and Arnold Palmer never straightened their legs, and they were some of the greatest shot makers and players in history.

To further clarify, the left knee anatomically must get at least over and above the left foot

Fig. 7.11 Premature straightening of the left leg

Fig. 7.12 Ben Hogan's soft knees allowed a smooth weight transfer.

before any kind of straightening occurs. As long as that happens, it doesn't matter what the left leg does. When the left knee gets over and on top of the left foot, you've got it!

Here is a set of sequenced flexibility exercises to allow your legs to maintain stability and mobility. (These drills are also applicable for straightening the legs on the backswing as indicated in Fault No. 1: Poor Address and Takeaway Problems.)

SUMMARY

All the drills and stretches recommended in this chapter will help you correct your golf swing faults and build a much more fundamentally sound swing, both physically and mechanically. They will help you to be able to do what you and your instructor are trying to accomplish in your swing.

The exercises connected with these specific drills should not be used as a substitute for your entire flexibility program, but rather as an addendum. Always regard your daily program (outlined in Chapter 10) as your main staple for flexibility conditioning and for better golf.

Golf Swing Drills

1. Left-leg-pivot drill (D14, page 110)

2. Pullback drill (D4, page 96)

Stretches

1. Single-leg pelvic tilt (S4, page 151)

2. Double-leg pelvic tilt (S5, page 151)

3. Straight-leg hamstring stretch (S8, page 153)

(continued)

Stretches—cont.

4. Adductor stretch
(S9, page 154)

5. Abductor stretch
(S10, page 154)

6. Psoas stretch
(S14, page 158)

7. Russian ball twist
(S34, page 175)

8. Quadriceps stretch
(S11, page 155)

9. Hip crossover
(S19, page 162)

CHAPTER
8

SWING FAULT SOLUTIONS

THIS CHAPTER CONTAINS DRILLS that are specific to different segments of the golf swing. The best way to utilize the drills is to practice them along with your flexibility program. As your flexibility improves, the drills will become more effective and definitely accelerate your progress to a freer and more powerful golf swing.

ADDRESS AND STABILITY DRILLS
D1. Close-the-Eyes Balance Drill

BENEFIT Practicing this drill, even during your round, will help you achieve a balanced address position.

STEP 1 Get into your address position while holding a golf club parallel to the ground (*Fig. 8.1*). Close your eyes and pay specific attention to where your weight is on your feet, e.g., heels, toes, balls of feet, insides, outsides.

Fig. 8.1 Weight 50-50 on each foot, with the majority on the balls of the feet

91

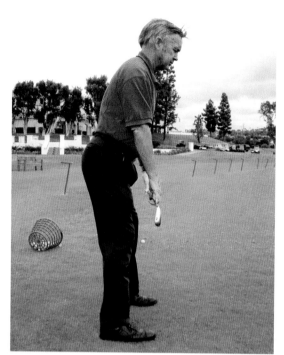

Fig. 8.2 Bend from your hips, allowing your arms to hang softly. The hip joint should be directly in line with the ankle.

STEP 2 Make sure your weight is 50-50 on each foot, and that the majority of your weight (about 60 percent) is on the balls of your feet with just a slight amount on the heels and toes *(Fig. 8.2)*.

Your arms should hang straight down and, if you let go of the club, it should land just in front of your toe line. If you do this drill without a club, clasp your hands. This will put you into perfect balance, and you'll be ready to go.

D2. Barefoot Balance Drill

BENEFIT Mastering this drill pays great dividends in your golf swing, because maintaining balance in the lower body will eliminate many swing faults that occur in the upper body.

STEP 1 Stand barefoot (on grass) in your address position, paying strict attention to where the weight and weight pressure are on your feet *(Fig. 8.3)*. Your weight should be 50–50 on each foot, with the majority on the balls of your feet.

STEP 2 Go ahead and swing. (You can hit a ball during this drill.) Pay attention to where the weight and weight pressure are on your feet during your swing. On the backswing, most of your weight should go onto the ball of your right foot *(Fig. 8.4)*, and on the forward swing, your weight should shift to the ball of your left foot *(Fig. 8.5)*, and then immediately toward your left heel *(Fig. 8.6)*. You'll be able to quickly determine if your weight distribution is in balance.

Fig. 8.3 Address position

Fig. 8.4 Weight on the ball of the right foot

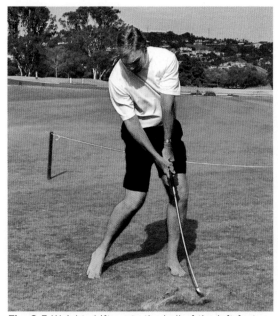

Fig. 8.5 Weight shifts onto the ball of the left foot

Fig. 8.6 Weight finishes on the left foot toward the heel

D3. **Foam-Roller Drill**

BENEFIT This outstanding drill helps eliminate excess rotation or sliding in your swing. You will need a half-round foam roller for this drill.

STEP 1 While barefoot, get into your address position on a half-round foam roller, making sure that you're perfectly balanced *(Fig. 8.7)*. Try not to let your toes or heels touch the ground. Depending on the size of the foam roller, they may touch; if so, keep your weight very light on your toes and heels.

STEP 2 Make some golf swings, feeling your weight shift onto the ball of your right foot *(Fig. 8.8)*, then back onto your left foot *(Figs. 8.9 and 8.10)*. Make sure that your hips turn as you shift onto your left foot, maintaining balance. You can also place an Impact Bag perpendicular to your left foot and swing into it *(Fig. 8.11)*.

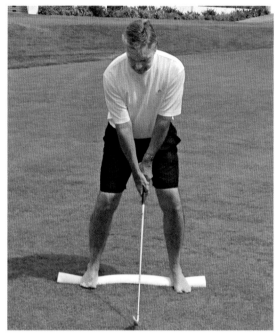

Fig. 8.7 Address position on half-round foam roller

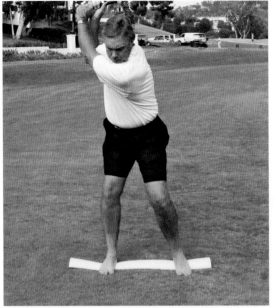

Fig. 8.8 Weight shifts onto the ball of the right foot

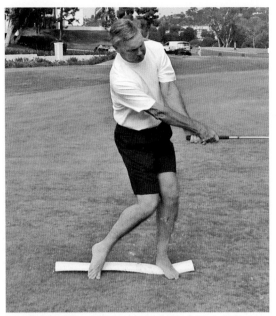

Fig. 8.9 Weight shifts onto the ball of the left foot

Fig. 8.10 Follow-through

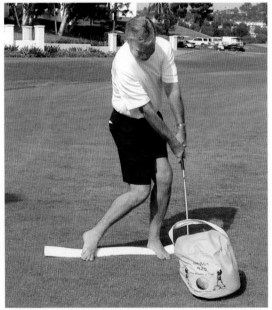

Fig. 8.11 Alternate: Impact Bag perpendicular to the left foot

D4. **Pullback Drill**

BENEFIT Mastery of this three-part drill helps eliminate excessive movements in the golf swing and helps develop lower-body stability. This is the most common and effective drill of all the drills I use.

STEP 1 Tee the ball up slightly with an 8 iron. Get into your address position and pretend that you're standing in dried concrete and that your legs are completely frozen *(Fig. 8.12)*.

STEP 2 On the backswing, swing the club upward while keeping your lower body as braced as possible *(Fig. 8.13)*. (Try to keep your belt buckle pointing at the ball.) I frequently videotape my students while they perform this drill, and they're always amazed at how much they've still turned and rotated at the top of their swings, since they feel that they haven't moved at all.

Fig. 8.12 Set up as if in dried concrete

Fig. 8.13 Backswing with lower body braced

STEP 3 From the top of your restricted backswing, swing your arms down through the ball and into the finish without moving your lower body *(Fig. 8.14)*. Make sure that you keep your right foot flat as you swing through.

STEP 4 From the finish of your arm swing, pull (swing) the shaft back to the original address position *(Fig. 8.15)*.

The secret of this drill is to keep the right foot flat on the ground throughout the entire swing. After hitting five good shots, you can graduate to part II of the pullback drill (D4A, page 98).

Fig. 8.14 Swing through the ball

Fig. 8.15 Backswing to the original address position

D4A. **Pullback Drill, Part II**

`STEP 1` For part II of the pullback drill, repeat steps 1 and 2 of part I *(Figs. 8.12 and 8.13).* (Remember to try not to turn your hips.)

`STEP 2` Instead of freezing your lower body as you swing down, go ahead and let your body release as you swing into a full finish. In other words, you can release your right foot now. Be sure to swing your arms all the way around with your right foot rising up onto its toe and your chest facing left of the target *(Fig. 8.16).* Repeat this drill until you hit five good shots. While performing this drill, think to yourself, "No backswing with the hips, and all forward swing."

Fig. 8.16 Right foot on its toe with chest facing left of target

D4B. **Pullback Drill, Part III**

After you've hit five good shots on parts I and II of this drill, now you are ready for part III *(Figs. 8.17–8.19).* This time, instead of keeping your torso as still as possible on the backswing, go ahead and shift your weight slightly onto the ball of your right foot and let your left shoulder come under your chin *(Fig. 8.18).* In other words, make a more normal backswing with your upper body (still keeping your lower body restricted), then swing down and through the shot into the finish *(Fig. 8.19).*

Fig. 8.17 Address position

Fig. 8.18 Weight shifted slightly onto the ball of the right foot

Fig. 8.19 Make a normal weight shift through the shot

D5. **Push-Away Drill**

`BENEFIT` This drill gets the weight shifting and the club moving back on a straight path. You will need a head cover, plastic water bottle, or any other suitable object for this drill.

`STEP 1` Get into your address position with a ball in front of you and a head cover or water bottle placed directly behind the clubhead *(Fig. 8.20)*.

`STEP 2` Sweep the object away as you move into your backswing *(Fig. 8.21)*. You'll feel a smooth weight shift onto your right foot.

Fig. 8.20 Address position with head cover behind clubhead.

Fig. 8.21 Sweep away the object.

D6. Elbow-to-Wall Drill

BENEFIT This drill focuses on the turn and helps teach you the uninterrupted flow you should feel in your upper trunk.

STEP 1 Stand 6 to 8 inches away from a wall or post. Make a fist with your left hand, letting your thumb stick out. Now point your thumb into the middle of your sternum *(Fig. 8.22)*.

STEP 2 Keeping your forearm level, simply turn your upper torso until your left elbow touches the wall, while making sure you stay in your spine angle *(Fig. 8.23)*. Make sure that the gap between your right thigh and the wall stays constant. In other words, don't let your right hip slide into the wall. (If it does, you probably have tight hips.)

Fig. 8.22 Thumb pointed into sternum

Fig. 8.23 Left elbow touching wall

Fig. 8.24 Place club shaft on right shoulder

Fig. 8.25 Turn shoulders

Fig. 8.26 Extend arms away from torso

D7. **Set, Turn, and Place Drill**

BENEFIT This drill synchronizes the arms, torso, and club, putting you into a balanced position at the top of your swing.

STEP 1 Stand in a balanced address position. While maintaining your posture and spine angle, simply fold your arms and set the club shaft on your right shoulder *(Fig. 8.24).*

STEP 2 Keeping the shaft on your shoulder and staying in your spine angle, make a relaxed shoulder turn *(Fig. 8.25).*

STEP 3 Extend your arms away from your torso *(Fig. 8.26).*

D8. **Baseball Drill**

BENEFIT This drill helps you develop a proper weight shift throughout your swing. This drill is especially helpful for people who have trouble shifting their weight properly in the takeaway.

STEP 1 Assume your address position *(Fig. 8.27)*. You're not going to hit the ball just yet.

STEP 2 Swing back and shift your weight onto your right foot. As you shift back, lift your left foot off the ground (toward your right knee) so

Fig. 8.27 Address position

Fig. 8.28 Weight shifted onto the right side, the left foot lifted

Fig. 8.29 Repeat steps 1 and 2 twice

that you're completely balanced on your right foot *(Fig. 8.28)*. Stay there for a moment, allowing your body to feel the balance point. Repeat this two times *(Fig. 8.29)*.

STEP 3 Keeping the feel of your weight shift onto your right foot, swing back again *(Fig.*

8.30). This time, keep your left foot down on the backswing and swing through into the finish *(Figs. 8.31 and 8.32)*. Once you get back to the right side and you're loaded and in balance, almost everything else is secondary. It happens almost automatically.

Fig. 8.30 Keep the left foot down

Fig. 8.31 Downswing, shifting weight to the left side

Fig. 8.32 Follow through

D9. Dick Mayer Drill

Dick Mayer, the winner of the 1957 U.S. Open and 1957 World Championship of Golf, taught me this drill. Mayer learned the drill from Ben Hogan when the two of them used to practice together in Fort Worth, Texas, in the fall, getting ready for the next year.

According to Mayer, Hogan hit thousands of balls using this drill. He would simply cock his wrists so that his left hand was opposite his right thigh and his shaft was parallel to the ground. From there, he would pump the club with a very restricted backswing and hit through the shot with an aggressive, full motion. Hogan told Mayer he wanted to eliminate any excessive length and overswinging in his backswing. When he first became a pro, Hogan had a long backswing and was often unable to control it. He tightened his backswing, and this drill was one way he kept it that way.

BENEFIT This is a great drill for eliminating excessive backswing movements.

STEP 1 Start by cocking your wrists so that the back of your left hand is directly opposite your right thigh, with the shaft parallel to the ground and parallel to the target line *(Fig. 8.33)*.

STEP 2 Pump the club slightly on the backswing *(Fig. 8.34)* and swing on through the shot *(Fig. 8.35)*.

Fig. 8.33 Hold shaft parallel to the ground

Fig. 8.34 Pump the club slightly

Fig. 8.35 Swing through the shot

D10. **Bruce Summerhays Drill**

I used to see Bruce start every practice session with this drill.

BENEFIT The upper body in the golf swing is a blending of a torso turn, an arm swing, and a wrist cock. Many golfers have difficulty blending all these elements together. This drill helps synchronize these body parts and will enable them to achieve a more fluid motion, particularly helping you feel the action of the wrists. Many people are intimidated to try this drill because they feel a lack of control with the club placed above the ball, but after doing it a couple of times they are usually amazed at how well they can hit the ball.

STEP 1 Start in your address position with the shaft fully cocked so that it's parallel to the ground and straight out in front of you *(Fig. 8.36)*.

STEP 2 Swing back and hit the ball *(Figs. 8.37 and 8.38)*.

Fig. 8.36 Hold shaft parallel to the ground

Fig. 8.37 Swing back

Fig. 8.38 Follow through

Fig. 8.39 Address position

Fig. 8.40 Stop at the top for a moment

Fig. 8.41 Follow through

D11. Stop-at-the-Top Drill

Even perfect mechanics won't do you any good if you don't have balance, rhythm, and timing. Undoubtedly, the most important move in the golf swing is the transition from the top of the swing down into impact. If you start down too soon with your hands or upper body at the top of the backswing, instead of allowing your lower body to initiate the downswing motion, the odds of hitting a good shot are greatly diminished.

BENEFIT This drill teaches you to overcome the temptation of starting down too quickly, and it helps you develop a slight pause at the top of the swing, which will enable your lower body to unwind first, thereby improving your rhythm and timing.

STEP 1 Address the ball *(Fig. 8.39)*.

STEP 2 Swing back to the top of your backswing and come to a complete stop *(Fig. 8.40)*. Hold it there for 2 seconds.

STEP 3 Return to the address position and repeat Step 2.

STEP 4 Make a normal swing *(Fig. 8.41)*. Now you'll feel the temptation to start down too soon, only it will be replaced by a nice hesitant pause at the top.

FORWARD-SWING DRILLS
D12. **Right-Arm-Only Drill**

BENEFIT This drill is designed to teach you the proper feel of shifting your weight and clearing your left side as you swing through the shot.

STEP 1 Take out a 6 iron or 7 iron, turn it upside down, and grip it just above the hosel with your right hand. Place the shaft behind you as if you were going to throw it down the fairway *(Fig. 8.42)*. This shouldn't be hard since many of us have probably done that after hitting a bad shot!

STEP 2 Swing the shaft forward *(Fig. 8.43)* and make the shaft *whoosh* on the front left side of your body *(Fig. 8.44)*. You should feel a smooth weight shift, release, and rotation through the motion.

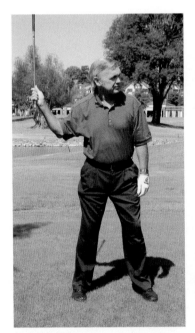

Fig. 8.42 Turn iron upside down and grip it just above the hosel

Fig. 8.43 Step forward while swinging the right arm

Fig. 8.44 Make the shaft *whoosh*

D12A. **Advanced Right-Arm-Only Drill**

The advanced right-arm-only drill is similar to the right-arm-only drill (D12, page 107), only now you're really going to hit a ball with your right arm only. Most golfers don't shift their weight to the left side and instead hang back, which keeps the center of gravity behind the ball and can create a swing that is out of control. Pay attention to how solidly you hit the ball. Solid is good.

STEP 1 Tee up a ball relatively low to the ground. Take a grip with your right hand, slightly choked down from your normal grip.

STEP 2 Place the club above and in front of the ball, with the shaft parallel to the ground *(Fig. 8.45).*

STEP 3 Swing back to the top *(Fig. 8.46)* and then back down, actually hitting the ball. The secret of success with this drill is to make a concentrated effort to shift your weight forward during the downswing *(Fig. 8.47).* If you don't shift your weight forward but instead hang back on your right side, this drill will be difficult to perform.

Fig. 8.45 Club shaft above and in front of the ball

Fig. 8.46 Swing back to the top

Fig. 8.47 Weight shifted forward

D13. Step-on-the-Gas Drill

Most golfers fail to shift their weight properly onto the left foot on the forward swing, instead either straightening the left leg too early or hanging back on the right foot. Doing either causes a golfer to lose power and consistency.

BENEFIT This drill helps you shift your lower body forward on the downswing. You'll probably find that paying more attention to the forward swing will automatically help put you into a better position on the backswing. Using a towel is optional for this drill.

STEP 1 Pretend that there's a gas pedal (accelerator) under your left foot. To get a better feel, you can take a towel or other flat object and place it underneath your left foot (Fig. 8.48).

STEP 2 As you start your downswing, "step on the gas" by trying to get 90 percent of your weight on the ball of the left foot before the club gets to the ball. To do this properly, start shifting your flexed left knee and hip onto your left foot, making sure you don't let your upper body move out in front as you do so (Fig. 8.49).

Fig. 8.48 Imaginary gas pedal under left foot

Weight Shifts Forward

Towel

Fig. 8.49 Left knee flexed until weight hits the left foot

D14. **Left-Leg-Pivot Drill**

BENEFIT This drill helps you feel the rotation of your hips and shoulders through the ball while stabilizing on a solid left side and also allows you to feel your right side release.

STEP 1 Get a 7 iron or 8 iron. Take an address position, with the ball slightly forward of middle in your stance. Drop your right foot behind you so that you're up on your toes and balancing primarily on your left leg *(Fig. 8.50).*

STEP 2 Swing back and through *(Figs. 8.51 and 8.52).* As you start down, consciously try to rotate your left hip and shoulder through the shot. You should almost feel that you're coming over the top with your shoulders, but you won't be because your left hip will be stabilized.

Fig. 8.50 Right foot on toes, balancing primarily on the left leg

Fig. 8.51 Swing back . . .

Fig. 8.52 . . . and through

D15. **Brush-the-Grass Drill**

BENEFIT This drill helps you develop the proper feel of your left side rotating out of the way as well as staying in your spine angle.

STEP 1 With no club in your hand, take your address position while placing your right arm away from your body *(Fig. 8.53)*. Let your left arm hang softly, or bring it up to your chest.

STEP 2 Simply swing down with your right hand and arm, imagining that you're going to brush the grass with your right hand *(Fig. 8.54)*.

Fig. 8.53 Backswing with the right arm away from body

Fig. 8.54 Swing down with the right arm as if trying to brush the grass

D16. **Wall-Press Drill**

`BENEFIT` This is a lower-body exercise. Mastery of it will do wonders for properly moving your lower body into the shot.

`STEP 1` Facing the corner of a wall or doorway, get into and address position and place your right hand on the wall so that your forearm is parallel to the floor and applying force into the wall *(Fig. 8.55)*. (Bare feet not necessary.)

`STEP 2` Firmly press your right hand and arm into the wall and apply extra pressure into the ball of your left foot while your right foot presses forward. You should also feel your thighs pressing, and you'll notice that your hips will automatically begin turning *(Fig. 8.56)*. You should feel a lot of torque on the outside of your left hip. This is precisely what the lower body should feel like as you shift and turn into the ball during your golf swing.

Fig. 8.56 Apply pressure in the feet, thighs, and hips

D17. **Power Fan Drill**

`BENEFIT` This drill helps strengthen your body, create power, and increase your two-cheek position. Combined with a flexibility program, swinging the fan is great training. You will need a power fan for this drill.

`STEP 1` Get into a proper address position while holding a power fan. While in your address position, cock your wrists and place the power fan just outside your right thigh with the fan approximately parallel to the ground and parallel to the target line *(Fig. 8.57)*.

`STEP 2` Pump the fan by going into a modified backswing *(Fig. 8.58)*, and then swing it through, making the fan *whoosh* in the front and on the left side of your body *(Figs. 8.59 and 8.60)*. The wings of the fan create wind resistance, and you're going to have to use some extra effort to really make it *whoosh*.

Fig. 8.55 Press the forearm and hand into the wall

Fig. 8.57 Hold power fan with your hands just outside your right thigh

Fig. 8.58 Modified backswing

Fig. 8.59 Swing the fan, creating a *whoosh*

Fig. 8.60 Swing the fan to the left of the target

D18. **Impact Bag Drill**

BENEFIT Swinging into an Impact Bag teaches the proper movement patterns of swinging into the ball. You will need an Impact Bag for this drill.

STEP 1 Take a normal address position with the club behind the Impact Bag *(Fig. 8.61)*.

STEP 2 Swing into the bag, making sure to shift your weight forward as you swing *(Fig. 8.62)*.

If you want to learn to draw the ball, simply turn the toe of the club into the bag as you swing into it; hold the clubface open for a soft fade.

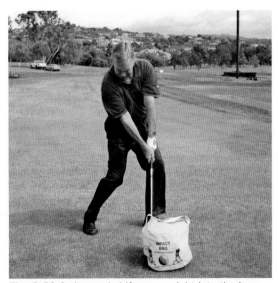

Fig. 8.61 Take a normal backswing

Fig. 8.62 Swing and shift your weight into the bag

Fig. 8.63 Towel underneath left armpit

Fig. 8.64 Rotate through the shot, keeping the towel tucked under your armpit

D19. Connection Drill

BENEFIT This drill is very effective in helping the arms work in sync with the torso. It is especially helpful in eliminating the dreaded chicken wing. You will need a towel or head cover for this drill.

STEP 1 Put a towel or head cover underneath your left armpit and set up in the address position *(Fig. 8.63)*.

STEP 2 Take some three-quarter swings, making sure that the towel stays tucked in your armpit *(Fig. 8.64)*. If the towel falls out, your swing has gotten too "arm-y." Make sure that you rotate your hips and shoulders through the shot as you swing through. Go ahead and hit balls with this drill.

Fig. 8.65 Flag on shoulders behind head with majority on right side

Fig. 8.66 Turning back

Fig. 8.67 Swing through making the flag *whoosh*

ROTATION DRILLS
D20. Flagstick Drill

BENEFIT This simple drill teaches the proper rotation of the hips and shoulders and helps maintain your spine angle throughout your swing. You will need a flagstick or long pole for this drill.

STEP 1 Place a flagstick on your shoulders behind your head. Make sure the flag and the majority of the pole are on the right side of your body *(Fig. 8.65)*.

STEP 2 Get into your address position and simply turn back *(Fig. 8.66)*. At the top of your backswing, the end of the flagstick should be pointing about 14 to 36 inches outside the imaginary ball. Swing through, making the flag *whoosh* at the same spot *(Fig. 8.67)*.

Fig. 8.68 Club across chest with clubhead parallel to spine and the toe facing upward

Fig. 8.69 Backswing

Fig. 8.70 Forward swing

D21. **Upper-Thorax Drill**

BENEFIT This simple drill teaches the proper shoulder rotation in the golf swing.

STEP 1 Place a 5 iron across your chest up around your shoulders *(Fig. 8.68)*. Make sure that the toe of the club is facing upward and the clubhead is parallel to your spine.

STEP 2 Hold the club in place and make a backswing *(Fig. 8.69)* and forward swing *(Fig. 8.70)*, imagining that you're hitting the ball with the head of the 5 iron.

DRILLS FOR ROUNDED SHOULDERS/ FORWARD HEAD POSTURE TYPES
D22. **Narrow the Stance Drill**

BENEFIT A wider stance tends to restrict movement, and since this posture type is indicative of restricted and tight muscles, I recommend a narrow stance. Doing so will allow your weight to shift easier and allow your body to rotate, thus not putting too much strain on your tight muscles.

STEP 1 Get into your address position, making sure that your feet are underneath your shoulders, or that the insides of your feet are parallel to the outsides of your shoulders *(Fig. 8.71)*.

STEP 2 Make sure that the majority of the weight is directly underneath the arches of your feet.

Fig. 8.71 Feet underneath shoulders

D23. **Stand Taller Drill**

BENEFIT The more that a person is bent over (as forward-head posture types are), the harder it is for the body to rotate and move. This means that when a person's chest muscles are tight, they won't be able to expand on the back and forward swing. Standing taller will help you move easier, and not force your body into unnecessary compensations. I can't stress this swing tip enough!

STEP 1 From a vertical and erect position, take your address position and bend ever so slightly from the hips, with the majority of your weight underneath the arches of your feet.

STEP 2 You should feel almost like you're standing straight up.

Fig. 8.72 Standing taller allows more freedom of motion . . . and balance.

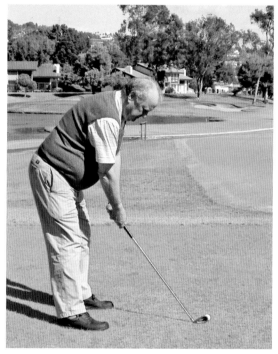

Fig. 8.73 A hunched-over address position

D24. **Strengthen the Grip Drill**

BENEFIT Because this posture type has restricted muscles, it's advisable to allow the hands to have more play in the swing. Strengthening both hands (turning to the right) will create more wrist action and help make up for the lack of function throughout your body.

STEP 1 Take your grip, making sure that the grip is down close to the roots of the fingers of your left hand. Turn your left hand over so that the V formed by your thumb and forefinger is pointed at least to your right shoulder.

STEP 2 Now take your right hand and set the "lifeline" of your right palm snugly over your left thumb. The thumb and forefinger of your right hand should be pointing at your right shoulder *(Fig. 8.74)*.

Fig. 8.74 A stronger grip makes it much easier to release the club.

DRILLS FOR C-CURVE/UNDER POSTURE

D24. Strengthen the Grip Drill

See page 119.

D25. Widen the Stance Drill

BENEFIT Although I generally don't prefer wide stances, we've got to get some lower-body stability into the C-curve posture's golf swing. By widening the stance, we'll create much needed stability in the foundation. This will also help curb the lifting that is almost sure to occur during the swing.

STEP 1 Take your normal address position with the ball positioned appropriately for the club you're using (that is, for a driver, position the

Fig. 8.75 A wider stance allows a more solid base of support.

ball just off your left heel; for a midiron, just slightly ahead of middle, and so forth).

STEP 2 Extend your right foot at least 6 more inches out to the right to widen your base. Make sure that the majority of your weight is directly under the arches of your feet (Fig. 8.75).

D7. Set, Turn, and Place Drill

See page 101.

DRILLS FOR ROTATED POSTURE

D26. Close Your Stance Drill

Right-handed golfers with a rotated posture have their hips and shoulders rotated to the left. This is normally due to having the right side dominant over the left from overuse. In the majority of cases, the rotated golfers will line up to the right because they kinesthetically feel squared that way.

BENEFIT One way to compensate for the rotation is to line up square, then draw your right foot back so that the right toe is parallel to the left heel. This will not only help square up the hips and shoulders, but it will also help keep the club on the inside, thus helping curb the club coming over the top.

STEP 1 From your address position, make sure that you're square to the target line (the line from the ball to the target).

STEP 2 Draw your right foot back so that the right toe is parallel to the left heel (Fig. 8.76).

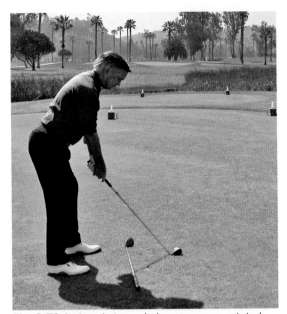

Fig. 8.76 A closed stance helps square up rotated hips and shoulders.

Fig. 8.77 Squaring up the left foot helps minimize a golfer from spinning out.

D27. Square Up Your Left Foot Drill

BENEFIT Having your left foot slightly flared out is not a bad thing, but with a rotated (to the left) posture you're actually enhancing and enabling the left hip to spin out even more. Keeping your left foot relatively square will make it a lot easier to get your left hip over onto your left side—thus encouraging a proper hip shift.

STEP 1 Take your address position.

STEP 2 Square your left foot so that your foot is perpendicular to the target line *(Fig. 8.77)*.

D28. Power Swing Left-Handed Drill

Because golfers with a rotated posture are so dominant on their right sides (in right-handers), we want to not only rid the body of the tight and imbalanced muscles but also eventually strengthen the left side.

BENEFIT Swinging the power fan left-handed (or any club for that matter) will help balance out both sides of the body, thus developing bilateral symmetry. You will need a power fan for this drill.

STEP 1 Take approximately 15 to 20 right-handed swings with the power fan.

STEP 2 Reverse the pattern and swing 15 to 20 times left-handed. You may be wondering, since you've overworked the dominant side for so many years, why not do more swings on the left? Simply reversing the pattern will help train

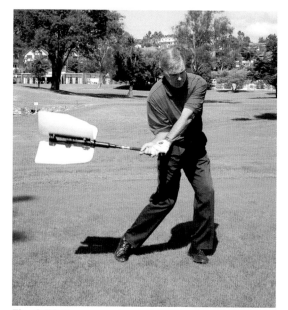

Fig. 8.78 See power fan drill (D17, page 112) and simply reverse and swing left-handed.

the left side to develop more neuron patterns, thus balancing out the body and reducing the right-side dominance.

D29. Hold Your Right Shoulder Back Drill

A rotated posture with the right shoulder lower and forward tends to force the club shaft out over the top, which in turn forces the left hip to spin out.

BENEFIT Holding the right shoulder back on the downswing not only helps keep the shaft from coming over the top but also forces the left hip to shift and get over to the left side.

STEP 1 After closing your stance, swing to the top of your backswing.

STEP 2 As you start down, try to hold your right shoulder back for as long as possible, making sure the club shaft stays to the inside.

Fig. 8.79 Holding the right shoulder back ensures an inside clubhead path.

CHAPTER

9

ANATOMY OF COMMON SWING THEORIES (AND OTHER MYTHS)

GOLF HAS MORE TIPS AND THEORIES than possibly all other sports combined, not to mention that many of them are contrary to one another. I've actually seen golf publications with conflicting tips from different golf professionals in the same issue. One such magazine had a swing tip that encouraged people to take the club back in a one-piece takeaway, while later in the same issue, another pro encouraged people to set the wrists early. Who is the reader to believe? It's no wonder this game has turned so many people into basket cases.

Yet, as we've discussed, nobody can definitively prove that their theory is really *the* correct theory for any individual. In all seriousness, as a teaching professional for years, I've lost track of the number of students who have gotten so obsessed and confused about this game that they

have gone to see a psychologist to get straightened out (which is interesting, because I've had several students that are shrinks, and a couple of them were just as confused as my other students).

Having studied the game from both the instruction side as well as the physiological side, I'd like to give a true, unbiased look at several common golf swing tips and theories from an anatomical perspective.

KEEPING THE HEAD STILL

This swing tip has been around since bored sheepherders began hitting rocks around the pasture with their crooks. Very few golfers in history actually kept their heads perfectly still, but a few of the all-time greats did.

123

These include Arnold Palmer, Jack Nicklaus, Bobby Jones, and Freddie Couples, to name a few. I've actually shown Arnold Palmer many videos of his swing throughout different periods of his career where his head did move, and he adamantly maintains that those videos were "bad" swings he just happened to make at the time. I do admit, however, that for most of his career he did keep his head still.

The truth is that the overwhelming majority of great players do move their heads. Since the head is connected to the spine, and the upper spine rotates over to the right side during the golf swing, it's only natural that the head rotates along with it *(Fig. 9.1)*. The Creator designed us to have two pivot points—a left and a right hip. By keeping the head still, the upper-body weight isn't allowed to shift

naturally into the right hip, therefore retarding an efficient weight transfer *(Fig. 9.2)*. Although keeping the head still does help prevent excess movement in the swing, a serious problem usually evolves: The weight is prevented from loading properly into the hips, thus putting a tremendous strain on the fascia in the lower back. Over time, this will usually lead to back pain. Golfers who keep their head still (e.g., Palmer, Nicklaus, and Couples) are more prone to back problems, and subsequently end up with back pain. When the weight is properly loaded into the hips, the friction is taken off the joint and thereby avoids straining other compensatory muscles and joints.

Fig. 9.1
A slight rotation of the upper spine and head allows a smooth weight transfer.

Fig. 9.2
Keeping the head still retards a proper weight shift.

KEEPING THE LEFT WRIST FLAT

There have been great players throughout history who played with cupped wrists *(Fig. 9.3)*, flat wrists *(Fig. 9.4)*, and even convex wrists *(Fig. 9.5)*. Most teachers, however, seem to prefer a flat left wrist.

The position of your wrist at the top of the swing normally depends on two factors: the thickness of the musculature around your wrists, and how you grip the club—either in a strong, weak, or neutral manner.

Generally speaking, people who are thick chested and on the chunky side tend to have flat or convex wrists at the top. Conversely, people who are slender and have skinnier wrists tend to cup their wrists a little more. As far as the grip, people who have a strong grip tend to create more cup in their left wrist, since the left

Fig. 9.3 Freddie Couples's cupped wrists

Fig. 9.4 Jack Nicklaus's flat wrists

Fig. 9.5 Dustin Johnson's convex wrists

hand is turned over to the right at a more pronounced angle, and is, in a sense, already somewhat cupped; golfers who have neutral or even weak grips tend to have their wrists flat.

Unless your hand position at the top is extreme one way or the other, or is causing you a lot of problems with the position of your clubface, I wouldn't worry about it very much.

UPRIGHT SWINGS OR FLAT SWINGS

Ben Hogan and Jack Nicklaus were the two greatest players of their time. Hogan had a flat swing plane *(Fig. 9.6)*, Jack an upright one *(Fig. 9.7)*. There has been a lot of controversy on which way is the best way. If one way was better than the other, then one of those guys was doing it wrong. I don't think so! Jim Hardy,

Fig. 9.6 Ben Hogan's flatter swing plane

Fig. 9.7 Jack Nicklaus's upright swing plane

who is a friend of mine, has created one of the most successful books and videos of the past decade, *The Plane Truth for Golfers*. Jim feels that, in theory, the one-plane swing is the most effective way to swing and, as a result, legions of golfers have switched over to that method. What is often overlooked is that Jim has also said that most people are better off using a two-plane swing, simply because to swing in one plane, one needs superb flexibility.

I agree with Jim that, in theory, a one-plane swing is probably the best way to go about it, but to get an efficient one-plane swing, a person has to have a much steeper shoulder plane during the turn. Hogan, for example, stood very tall at address and dipped down quite a bit, which made it easier to get his left arm in line with his shoulder plane. In other words, the more the left shoulder goes down, the easier it is for the left arm to get on plane. Arnold Palmer also turned his shoulders on a steep angle, and he was probably the poster boy for the one-plane swing. However, the more the shoulders flatten out, the harder it is to get the arms on plane with them, and instead they'll tend to lift up.

What I'm saying is that since most people don't possess enough flexibility to tilt their shoulders deeply, they therefore shouldn't be trying to do something their bodies can't do effectively.

In summary, people who are more slender and possess ample flexibility can give the one-plane swing a try. Shorter, stockier people who are not very flexible are usually better off using a two-plane system.

KEEPING THE RIGHT FOOT FLAT THROUGH IMPACT

A fairly common swing tip in recent years has been to keep the right foot flat through impact. This has become popular with the evolution of the modern swing, where many teachers emphasize less leg action. The reason behind this is an effort to curb the player from driving the legs too much, which usually gets the clubhead stuck behind him. This is accurate, but I think this swing tip should be reserved for Tour players and better golfers. Tour pros play a lot of shots in the wind, and as a result, often get into the habit of driving into the shot too much; that is, trapping the ball. Plus, the modern swing incorporates a narrower stance, so there's much less need or room to drive the legs.

For the average player, in fact for many golfers, it's not a good road to travel. The main difference between Tour players and average high handicappers is that Tour players get to their left sides *(Fig. 9.8)* and high handicappers stay stuck back on their right sides *(Fig. 9.9)*, which inevitably leads to a hand flip through the ball. It doesn't make much sense to try to get high handicappers to keep their right foot flat when they're already stuck on their back foot.

For decades, one of the most successful swing tips, made especially popular by the "Silver Scot," Tommy Armour, was to kick the right knee and foot in toward the ball to start the downswing. For years, Gary Player would actually walk through to the target by taking a step down the fairway, and he certainly is one of the greatest players who ever lived.

Another reason the right foot comes off the ground is that the left hip pulls it off due to its

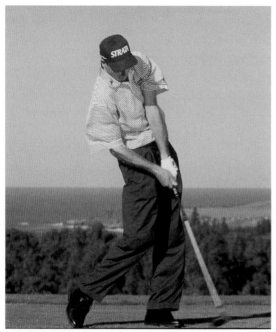

Fig. 9.8 Jim Furyk releasing his right side

Fig. 9.9 High handicapper stuck on right side

rotation through the shot. Thus, players endanger stunting their hip rotation by anchoring down that right foot.

Unless you're good enough to really work your shots like a Tour player, my advice is to let that foot go!

RETURN TO THE ADDRESS POSITION AT IMPACT

This swing tip is one of my all-time pet peeves. Many teachers taught it to me throughout the years, mainly in the 1960s and 1970s. Unfortunately, I actually believed it and got to the point where I perfected it!

Most instructors now know better. This the-

ory stated that at impact the hips and shoulders should be parallel to the target line, approximating where they were at address. After video cameras proved that the hips and shoulders were clearly open at impact *(Figs. 9.10 and 9.11)*, many teachers jumped on the bandwagon and conceded that the hips should be cleared but that the shoulders should remain square, or parallel to the target line. I once read where one world-renowned instructor actually wanted the buttons of one's shirt to aim right of the ball at impact! During one of my seminars on anatomical function in the golf swing at one of his golf schools, this instructor had me removed from the stage because he felt that I was preaching blasphemy when I explained how the hips and shoulders must be open at impact to create centrifugal force.

The fear that instructors have about allowing their students to have their shoulders open at impact is that by condoning this they feel that this will encourage golfers to come over the top. This is a very valid concern, but what really is responsible for clearing the shoulders is the rotation of the left hip. As explained in Chapter 3, in order to get the hips to turn properly, the lower body must shift over to the front foot first. The lateral shifting of the weight actually drops the club shaft into the slot before the shoulders have cleared. If the left knee, leg, and hip are solidly on the left foot and have gotten there first, you can't turn your shoulders enough!

Even as recently as this year, I've had vigorous debates with instructors who have told me that the shoulders still need to be square at impact, even while they were looking at videos that clearly showed that every great player's hips and shoulders were open at impact. When I pointed this out to them on video, their excuse was that the modern-day Tour player doesn't swing like that anymore. The player we were looking at was none other than Tiger Woods, so perhaps they figured that Tiger—and every great player and ball striker in history—has been doing it wrong!

Thanks to 3-D motion-capture systems, we've been able to quantify this position and have definite ranges that apply to the overwhelming majority of Tour players. On irons at impact, the hips of Tour players range from 35 to 50 degrees open, and the shoulders vary from 26 to 34 degrees open. (And for the record, we don't measure the shoulders from the actual clavicles—because the shoulder joints are movable joints, where one shoulder

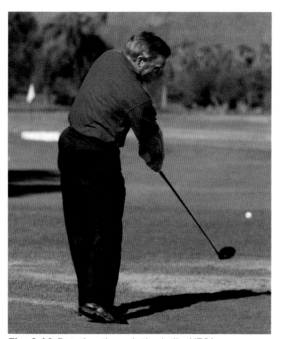

Fig. 9.10 Rotating through the ball—YES!

Fig. 9.11 Return to the address position—NO!

joint is likely to be rounded or forward—but rather from the T3 vertebra, in the upper back, just below where the spine connects with the neck). With drivers, the ranges are very similar, and in many cases even more open.

To prove this, simply pick up a baseball bat or a tennis racket and make a few swings, then take an object like a rock or baseball and throw it underhand-sidearm. Notice how your left hip and shoulder naturally shift and clear out of the way and allow a nice free follow-through of your arms. Now make some swings (or throws), only this time don't let your hips and shoulders open but keep them parallel to the target line. You'll notice that when you don't clear your hips and shoulders, your arms jam up. It won't take long for you to determine which of these methods is the proper action.

If anyone ever tells you to return to the address position at impact with your hips and shoulders square to the target line, run for the hills! The only thing that should return to the address position at impact is the clubface.

DEALING WITH FLYING ELBOWS

This swing "fault" has been around forever and has always been considered taboo. Thousands of golfers have practiced with handkerchiefs under their right armpit or straps around the upper arms to keep their arms connected.

Then came Jack Nicklaus with a flying right elbow. Flying elbows can be a bad thing, but they can also be a good thing if they're indigenous to your body type. Just ask Jack, Freddie Couples *(Fig. 9.12)*, Jim Furyk, Miller Barber, and legions more. It depends on how you're

built. Most flying elbows are symptomatic of tight chests and shoulder blades, or a "frozen scapula," as it's often called. In other words, people who have thick chests, backs, and shoulders tend to be more restricted than slender people. As their upper torso rotates in the backswing, if the muscles around the shoulder blades (traps, rhomboids, etc.) are tight, this condition will usually cause the arms to lift and become disconnected from the torso. To some degree this is okay, unless the arms begin to interrupt the natural rotation of the torso and then disconnect. This lifting also tends to unload the hips as they become destabilized by straightening the leg, overturning, or sliding.

Fig 9.12 A flying right elbow certainly hasn't hindered Freddie Couples.

One thing you don't want to do in the golf swing is lose your lower-body stability. However, if you maintain the stability in your lower body and your arms and elbows don't compromise your torso function, let your elbow go where it wants to. Allowing the spine and thorax to rotate easily and without interruption is absolutely crucial, so as long as your trunk is in control, let your elbows do what they want to do.

Regarding the forward swing, one place where you don't want your elbows to fly is right after impact, creating a chicken wing, where your left arm doesn't refold and swing into a full finish. A chicken wing means that the torso didn't release properly, the arms didn't release properly, and the wrists didn't release properly, in sequence.

In the case of chicken wings, or disconnection of the arms and elbows through the ball, I do recommend putting a head cover, handkerchief, or towel under the left armpit to practice rotating the torso through the ball with the upper left arm tucked to the side. (For a drill on this, see D19 on page 114). Another option is to tie a strap around the torso and upper left arm but let the right arm go where it wants. This will create some extra width with your right arm on the backswing yet keep your elbows from separating through the shot. To make this clear, I don't like straps or props on the right arm during the backswing, but I do recommend them on the left arm for the forward swing. Remember though, these drills should come after or with your flexibility program.

THE FLEXIBILITY AND STRENGTH PROGRAMS

JUST STRETCHING WON'T MAKE YOU FLEXIBLE

One of the great myths that I've discovered is that the majority of people think that stretching makes you flexible. I can assure you that stretching on its own won't make you flexible. Over many years, I have seen virtually thousands of people perform their stretching routines, and seldom have I seen these people actually become flexible! That was certainly true in my case. For years I stretched all the time, and not only did I not achieve superb flexibility, but I actually ended up injuring myself in the process.

I know now that I'm not alone in this because, for many years, my staff and I have asked thousands of students who have come to our golf schools if they stretch, and the vast majority of them have told us that they do. Yet, seldom have we seen very many flexible people!

This tells me that there is something wrong with this axiom because, if people stretch properly, they will increase the range of motion in their muscles, enhance the oxygenation of their bodies, rehabilitate injuries, and even prevent injuries from happening in the first place. As mentioned, the vast majority of people that I talk to don't receive these benefits. By deduction, it means that most people are stretching incorrectly. I have learned there is a right way to stretch and a wrong way to stretch. Let me explain the right way to stretch so that you can reap the many benefits that being flexible has to offer.

There are three rules that must be followed to achieve these benefits.

1. Breathe properly
2. Work the muscle chains in sequence
3. Maintain consistency in your practice

Most flexibility programs fail because one or more of the rules hasn't been followed.

RULE 1: **BREATHE PROPERLY**

When we stretch, we're not just stretching, we're actually breathing oxygen into the nerve spindles and nerve fibers throughout our muscles and into the fascia (a fibrous connective tissue that envelops, separates, or binds a muscle together). Within the fascia are thousands of nerve spindles and nerve fibers that connect with our nervous systems and go into our brains.

As we begin contracting and expanding a muscle, the fascia becomes pulled apart, so to speak, and as it stretches, the nerve spindles and nerve fibers of the muscle become separated from oxygen. As this happens, the nerves cry out to the brain, and we suddenly feel a burn. The burn is, in effect, a warning signal or a cry for help from the brain saying, "We need more oxygen down there!" If the cries for oxygen are ignored, the muscle can tear. The right way to stretch is to start the process of deep breathing and sending oxygen down into the nerve spindles and nerve fibers. As the oxygen flows into the fascia, the nerves begin to bathe in a sea of oxygen and relax. They then say to the muscle, "It's okay now. You can go ahead and contract and expand a little further." As a result, the muscle increases its range of motion and becomes flexible. If, however, the demand for oxygen isn't met, the muscle will tighten up,

a process called the myotatic reflex, or the stretch reflex. In order to protect itself, the brain signals an impulse down into the stressed area that tightens up the muscle, which is exactly what we don't want to happen. We want to relax the muscles, not tighten them. A flexible muscle is a relaxed muscle—nothing more, nothing less. And a relaxed muscle is one that has oxygen in it.

Not only does the oxygenating of our muscles stretch those muscles, our entire body receives the benefits of breathing. The diaphragm will help push the oxygen and blood into the heart, the heart then pumps the oxygen and blood throughout the body, and even more important, the head will begin to sit right on top of the shoulders. I encourage you to stand up right now and try that. Inhale and exhale deeply; notice how, on the inhalation, the chest not only expands but also pushes your head back on top of your shoulders. When the head sits right on top of the clavicles, gravity is allowed to circulate the oxygen and blood to nourish the brain. Nearly all people who embark on my flexibility program report back that they begin to feel taller and lighter and that they focus more clearly. This is from the increase in oxygen and blood to the brain due to the body becoming better balanced with improved posture. When something is better balanced, it actually will be lighter due to its alignment with gravity. Since we're actually doing over 20,000 repetitions of breathing a day, you can see how important breathing is. In time, developing proper breathing patterns will strengthen your body, and emotions, in a number of ways. The body's breathing pattern will begin to sustain itself.

Although there are a lot of different breathing techniques, I've narrowed it down to two methods that I employ in my stretching programs. I'm going to teach you a breathing method for the static stretches and a method for the active stretches. For the static stretches, we're going to employ east-west breathing and for the active stretches, we're going to reverse the process.

Static Stretches

For static stretches, where we hold the pose for 20 to 40 seconds, I want you to inhale through the nose, making sure that you expand your lower abdomen in a side-to-side manner. This breathing, called east-west, ensures that we employ intra-abdominal pressure into the solar plexus, which will, among other things, help to stabilize the spine. Imagine you have an inner tube fit snugly around your midsection, just under your rib cage. As you inhale, try to expand the entire inner tube outward. Or, as I like to say, "Get fat" by allowing your love handles to go outward. (We men sometimes find ourselves sucking it in in an effort to impress the ladies down at Muscle Beach.) To effectively breathe east-west, I want you to give up your ego and let it out. My experience has shown me that very few people can effectively perform east-west breathing in the beginning.

To test this breathing method, have someone put their fingers on the sides of your abdomen (where your love handles are), and as you breathe in, push out against your helper's fingers *(Fig. 10.1).* I've found that few people can do this very well in the beginning. However, by being conscious of this even while walking around during the day, you'll begin to breathe

powerfully and effectively. In time you'll find yourself breathing this way automatically, and at that point you'll find that it has a very calming and confident effect on your state of well-being.

Although the upper chest will also expand, the emphasis and focus should be on the lower abdomen. A huge mistake in people's breathing occurs when they just breathe with their upper chest in a panting manner, which is, in fact, actually a form of holding their breath.

At the end of the inhalation, I want you to actually feel a tightening up, or a pushing out, at your sides until they're firm. This is important to attain the "contract-relax" response that we want. Only tighten your sides at the end of the stretch, not before. This will be easier to do in certain postures and more difficult in others. At the end of the inhalation, pause for a moment, keeping tight, then exhale out through your mouth, making sure that you completely empty your entire solar plexus. (At this point, your abdomen will be collapsing back inward.)

Fig. 10.1 As you inhale, push outward against the fingers

On exhalation out through the mouth, the breath should sound like a *Haaaah*. This point is crucial in the process because this is when the total relaxation occurs. You'll notice that as you're exhaling you'll immediately go deeper and deeper into the stretch. This contract-relax process is very powerful and is sure to enhance your overall breathing capacity.

The main point here is to make sure that your inhalation and exhalation patterns are full and deep. In other words, don't cut off the inhalation or exhalation until you've reached the very end of the breath. You'll probably notice that if you try to force a stretch, you won't be able to sustain your breathing pattern and will instead be forced to hold your breath. If this happens, it is simply a sign that you're going too far at this point in the stretch and you are actually increasing tension. And tension is exactly what we *don't want!* Be patient and allow the breathing patterns to take you deeper into the stretch.

Let's review: (1) You want to inhale through the nose, making sure that you're pushing the sides of your lower abdomen outward (at the love handles) until they're firm; (2) at the end of the inhalation, hold for a moment; and (3) exhale completely through the mouth allowing all of the breath out of the lower abdomen. Pause and then repeat.

Active Stretches

On active stretches, the breathing pattern is the opposite of the east-west pattern. In this case, we're going to exhale out through the mouth on the first phase and then inhale in through the nose on the release. In addition, we're only going to hold the stretch for 1 to 2 seconds.

Nearly everybody I train has trouble coordinating this at first, so I tell them to think of baseball. Think of the first out. Breathe out on the first move, and inhale on the release.

Holding the pose for only 1 to 2 seconds prevents any chance of a stretch reflex. This is a tightening of the muscle, in essence shutting it down. Because you're holding the stretch for such a short time, there's no chance of any excess tightening of the muscle. Active stretches will also, in time, strengthen the fast-twitch fibers of the muscle.

There is much controversy about whether active stretches or static stretches are better for you. Advocates for active stretches say that static stretches and breathing slow down the fast-twitch fibers in the muscle, which make you slower and increase the wear and tear of the fascia because you're holding the muscle for a long time, day after day, month after month, year after year. This is very common in ballet dancers, who hold poses in awkward positions for years and commonly end up with a multitude of serious injuries.

In my experience, however, I have found that for rehabilitating muscle and improving one's posture, a static stretch is superior to an active stretch because the muscle fibers have more time to receive oxygen while they're in proper position and, therefore, the brain has more time to remember the proper neuron pattern. An active stretch is superior for sports where you're trying to improve speed and quickness, such as running and jumping. However, if one includes resistance training and cardiovascular with their static stretch program, their fast-twitch fibers will be just fine—and will allow them to develop a lot of speed and power!

In my programs, I use the best of both worlds and employ both methods.

RULE 2: **WORK THE MUSCLE CHAINS IN SEQUENCE**

Muscles work in chains. Much like tile on a roof, although they're all individual, muscles all work in unison and synergize with one another. There are several chains of muscles in our bodies, but the ones that we're going to be concerned with here are the posterior chain (the muscles on our back side that run from our heels up to our necks) and the anterior chain (three major muscles on the front of our hips that intertwine with the diaphragm). The muscles in these chains that have the most influence are called polyarticular (muscles that cross over two joints) and are on both sides of the body. When one muscle in the chain is shortened, the entire chain is affected, shortening the rest of the chain with it.

For example, the calf muscles in the posterior chain work in unison with the hamstrings, glutes, trapezii, etc. If, for example, a person has a tight calf, almost invariably we'll see a tight back or shoulder. Therefore, if I want to stretch out my back, I'll definitely need to stretch out the rest of the muscles in that chain, such as my calves, hamstrings, glutes, etc. If I only stretch my shoulders and neglect the other muscles in the chain, in a short amount of time the other tight muscles that weren't stretched will again pull the shoulders out of position. Simply isolating and stretching just one aspect of the chain will not make for permanent results.

Isolating and stretching individual muscles without stretching out the other muscles in the chain is probably the number one mistake (along with improper breathing) that the average person makes in their stretching.

It's important to work the muscle chains in order, from the ground up. Don't worry—you won't need to learn all of the muscle chains. The programs in this book are arranged for the muscles to be stretched in order, and in their respective chains. If you do the stretches in sequence, you'll be working the proper muscle chains in the proper order.

RULE 3: **MAINTAIN CONSISTENCY IN YOUR PRACTICE**

Consistency is extremely important. I stress this because our sedentary/sitting-down lifestyle tightens us up to some degree every day. Every day that we sit down we're "exercising" our hips in a flexed position, and therefore I feel that we must all incorporate a proper flexibility program into our daily lives to counterbalance the damaging effects of this lifestyle. Since most golfers, and especially our senior players, have tightened up as a result of this lifestyle, the majority of them must "build up," so to speak, to attain a flexible and functional body. It's better to be consistent and do a little bit every day than it is to do a lot 2 or 3 days a week. But don't shortchange yourself. If you're not making the strides that you're hoping for, you're probably not doing enough. Also, the more diligent and consistent you are in the beginning, the faster you'll attain results.

In the beginning, most of you aren't in a

position to just do it once in a while. Think of these programs as if you were going to train for a marathon. If you just went for a jog every few days, there's no way that you'd develop the endurance necessary to finish 26.2 miles. By working your programs on a consistent basis and then resting occasionally, you'll eventually build up enough endurance to finish the race and achieve superb flexibility. That's the best way to approach flexibility training.

I'm sure you're thinking, "Oh, no. I've got to do this forever." Don't fret, because I have some good news: The more flexibility you attain, the more you can maintain. In other words, you won't have to do as much because the more you train your body to breathe throughout your muscle chains, the more your body will learn how to breathe on its own, thus developing a stronger diaphragm and creating intra-abdominal pressure. Subsequently, your daily flexibility program certainly won't take very long. I've been stretching properly for more than 30 years, and my daily program now takes me around 10 minutes. When I started, however, it took me around 20 to 40 minutes. I assure you, it's been well worth it.

My goal with my clients is to get them to incorporate their flexibility programs into their daily lives, just like brushing their teeth. I highly recommend that you do your program 5 or 6 days a week, always taking one day off to allow your body to completely rest.

Don't rush into the program and burn out, either. Remember, the tortoise won the race, not the hare.

WHEN TO STRETCH Any time is a good time to stretch, but the morning is best because you're preparing the muscles for all the activity you're going to encumber during the day. Doing short stretches throughout the day (especially the psoas stretch—see S14, page 158) is also beneficial for restoring range of motion and energy. If you want to do some stretches at night, go right ahead.

WARM UP BEFORE STRETCHING It's a good idea to warm up before you stretch. You can do a little running in place, swing the power fan, or do any other cardio exercise for a few minutes. Heat in the body is what we're striving for, so a little warmup is good. You'll find, too, that the deeper and longer you breathe, the more you'll heat up and perspire. In the Advanced Program, a warmup is not that crucial because the active stretches themselves warm you up.

WARM UP BEFORE OTHER EXERCISE PROGRAMS You should always stretch before any exercise program. Ideally, do the entire stretch program. However, if you're short on time, then the Pregolf Warmup will suffice. You can do the Postgolf Cooldown when you're finished, or the relaxation poses.

HYDRATION Drink purified water before, during, and after your workout. This will help your oxygen and blood circulation as you work through your program.

THE PROGRAMS

There are three basic programs: the Short Program for beginners, the Intermediate Program, and the Advanced Program. I've also included the Pregolf Warmup as well as the Postgolf Cooldown, which are important as the muscles should be warmed before we play and unwound after play.

The Short Program and Intermediate Program incorporate static stretches, where you'll hold the poses for 20 to 40 seconds. These poses are designed to synchronize the muscle chains, increase oxygenation in your body, and help restore better posture.

The Advanced Program incorporates active stretches, where you only hold each pose for 1 to 2 seconds. This program is most beneficial for people who want to do more active forms of exercise, such as cardio training, basketball, tennis, and so forth. And yes, you can use it before you play golf, too.

Although I've coined these programs as beginner, intermediate, and advanced, it's perfectly okay to work all of them.

Relaxation Poses

I cannot stress relaxation poses enough! You should do them as much as possible. The supine groin stretch (S54, page 193) is the most effective pose that I've ever seen in taming the powerful hip flexors, especially the iliopsoas. Relaxing the psoas is critical because it's connected to the diaphragm, not to mention that it interacts with the sympathetic nervous system (which controls your fight-or-flight response). Every breath you take involves the hip flexors, and every step you take involves the hip flexors and diaphragm. I highly recommend that you take 1 or 2 days off a week and just do the supine groin stretch, even up to an hour or more if you can. This was the pose that convinced me of the importance of flexibility training and changed my life. Many people feel that the supine groin stretch isn't doing anything while they're in the pose, but I assure you it is. Relaxing the hips is absolutely crucial in devel-

oping anatomical function and allowing your body to return to proper posture. Once the hip flexors are relaxed, every muscle in the body is affected, and they will be closer to doing the job nature assigned them to do.

Mixing Up Your Programs

Mix up the programs. After all, doing the same program every day can get monotonous and cause you to burn out from boredom. After you master the programs, combine different parts of the different programs into one.

For example, let's say you do the Short Program's lower-body stretches, but you want to get more aggressive with the spinal twists. Go ahead and do the upper-body stretches in the Advanced Program. Or, you can do the active stretches for the lower body first and then do some static stretches for the upper body next.

The main thing to remember if you mix up your stretch programs is to always start from the ground up and always stretch the lower body first. In other words, don't start with the upper body, especially the spinal twists.

In an effort to get more flexible in their upper trunk so they can get a bigger shoulder turn, many people start right off on their spinal twists and don't do anything else. If you want more shoulder turn, loosen up the hips more! I've seen a lot of people increase their shoulder turns up to 40 degrees just by loosening their hips. In most cases, an inflexible muscle group can be loosened up just by stretching the other end of that muscle chain.

Injuries

The programs in this book were not designed to treat specific injuries. They were designed to increase the range of motion in a person's body to create a freer and more powerful golf swing. I am continually asked if this program will help this or that condition, and I normally reply that proper flexibility programs can help nearly all conditions—if the stretches are done and conducted in the proper sequence. However, all stretching protocols must be designed for that specific injury. If you have an injury, first see a licensed physician or anatomical functionalist before you go any further.

If you feel some pain when doing a stretch, stop that stretch immediately but continue to do the other stretches in the order prescribed.

Now that you know the rules, let's get into the programs.

SHORT PROGRAM

Note: A detailed explanation for each of the stretches in these programs can be found in Chapter 11. Each stretch has a corresponding reference and page number to assist in finding the detailed explanation.

1. Overhead extension (S35, page 176)

2. Counter (S22, page 165)

3. Cats and dogs (S23, page 165)

4. Downward dog (S1, page 149)

5. Psoas stretch (S14, page 158)

Or standing psoas stretch (S14A, page 158)

6. Spread-foot forward bend (S2, page 150)

7. Runner's stretch (S3, page 150)

8. Sitting wall
(S16, page 159)

9. Bridge (S24, page 166)

10. Pretzel
(S31, page 172)

11. Crocodile
(S33, page 174)

12. Cats and dogs
(S23, page 165)

13. Pectorals stretch
(S36, page 177)

14. Arm circle (S37, page 178)

15. Elbow curl
(S38, page 180)

INTERMEDIATE PROGRAM

1. Overhead extension
(S35, page 176)

2. Counter
(S22, page 165)

3. Cats and dogs
(S23, page 165)

4. Cobra
(S25, page 166)

5. Downward dog
(S1, page 149)

6. Plank
(S44, page 186)

7. Psoas stretch
(S14, page 158)

8. Triangle
(S26, page 167)

9. Extended lateral
(S27, page 168)

10. Spread-foot forward
bend (S2, page 150)

11. Runner's stretch
(S3, page 150)

12. Solo sitting wall
(S17, page 160)

13. Hip-thigh extension
(S18, page 161)

14. Hip crossover
(S19, page 162)

15. Pretzel
(S31, page 172)

16. Upper spinal floor
twist (S32, page 173)

–OR–

17. Extended half bow
(S28A, page 169)

17. The bow
(S28, page 169)

18. Why me
(S39, page 181)

19. Breaststroke
(S40, page 182)

20. Arm circle
(S37, page 178)

21. Elbow curl
(S38, page 180)

22. Air bench
(S51, page 192)

23. Static back press
(S53, page 193)

ADVANCED PROGRAM

1. Single-leg pelvic tilt (S4, page 151)

2. Double-leg pelvic tilt (S5, page 151)

3. Bent-knee hamstring stretch (S6, page 152)

4. Straight-leg hamstring stretch (S8, page 153)

5. Adductor stretch (S9, page 154)

6. Abductor stretch (S10, page 154)

7. Quadriceps stretch (S11, page 155)

8. Psoas stretch (S14, page 158)

Or standing psoas stretch (S14A, page 158)

9. Solo sitting wall (S17, page 160)

10. Hip-thigh extension (S18, page 161)

11. Internal and external hip rotators (S20, page 163)

12. Seated forward bend (S29, page 170)

13. Russian ball twist (S34, page 175)

Or pretzel (S31, page 172)

14. Locust (S50, page 191)

Or extended locust (S50B, page 191)

15. Lateral ball roll (S41, page 183)

16. Frog (S21, page 164)

17. Internal and external shoulder rotators (S42, page 184)

18. Why me (S39, page 181)

19. Breaststroke (S40, page 182)

20. Head and neck stretches (S43, page 185)

21. Wall squat (S49, page 190)

PREGOLF WARMUP

1. Overhead extension
(S35, page 176)

2. Counter (S22, page 165)

3. Cats and dogs
(S23, page 165)

4. Downward dog
(S1, page 149)

5. Psoas stretch
(S14, page 158)

6. Runner's stretch
(S3, page 150)

7. Pretzel
(S31, page 172)

8. Arm circle (S37, page 178)

9. Elbow curl
(S38, page 180)

POSTGOLF COOLDOWN

1. Overhead extension (S35, page 176)

2. Counter (S22, page 165)

3. Cats and dogs (S23, page 165)

4. Downward dog (S1, page 149)

5. Crocodile (S33, page 174)

6. Cats and dogs (S23, page 165)

7. Static back press (S53, page 193)

RELAXATION POSES

1. Cats and dogs
(S23, page 165)

2. Downward dog
(S1, page 149)

3. Static back press
(S53, page 193)

4. Supine groin stretch
(S53, page 193)

POWERFUL POSES FOR STRENGTH

Although this book is primarily about increasing your flexibility to improve your golf swing, it must be emphasized that resistance and cardiovascular training must also be included in any complete fitness program. However, I believe strongly that there must be an order to any proper fitness program.

My philosophy has always been to:

1. Relax the body

2. Increase the range of motion

3. Add on resistance and cardiovascular protocols . . . in that order.

Frankly, I've seen way too many people with dysfunctional bodies that are out of posture incorporate strengthening programs while their bodies were out of alignment. In many of these cases, the person has actually strengthened their dysfunctions and ended up becoming injured. Too many times I've had people come to me saying, "Roger, I just don't get it. I go to the gym all the time, yet it seems like I'm always hurt."

As I mentioned regarding the dangers of isolating muscle groups, the same applies to strength training. Just strengthening isolated parts of the body can end up creating imbalances, compensations, and eventually pain—not to mention causing the body to become anatomically dysfunctional. On this point, dysfunctional people are sometimes people who work out the most. Heavy power lifters usually have very little range of motion. (You know, the guys who can barely comb their hair because of their overloaded and bulky muscles.) In my opinion, this type of training is excellent for opening up pickle jars and catching the eyes of the ladies down at Muscle Beach, but is nearly always ineffective when it comes to hitting a golf ball. Again, when a muscle is overused, it loses its length-tension capacity and begins to shorten, and a short muscle doesn't move as well as a muscle that elongates. Therefore, I say that in reality a muscle that can't move . . . is a weak muscle.

Having said that, there are a lot of exercises that work the entire body and give a good stretch at the same time. Generally speaking, I prefer these whole-body strengthening exercises over strengthening isolated muscle groups any day.

The exercises that I present here should help work most or all of the major muscle groups in your body, thus allowing you to achieve a more functional body and golf swing.

I encourage you to incorporate this program into your routine at least 3 days a week.

In conjunction with the flexibility programs in this book, this short but effective routine will certainly help make your golf swing not only more fluid but also more powerful. And any extra yards certainly won't hurt when you play today's longer golf courses.

THE STRENGTH PROGRAM

Although I recommend that these strengthening exercises be done in this order, any or all of them may be done separately, because we're recruiting most, if not all of the muscles in the body's chains.

Although you can do these strengthening exercises anytime, I personally like to do them after my flexibility programs.

1. Cats and dogs (S23, page 165)

2. Baby dolphin (S46, page 188)

3. Dolphin (S47, page 188)

4. Triceps dip (S45, page 187)

5. Hand-leg opposite lift (S48, page 189)

6. Powerful air bench (S52, page 192)

7. Triceps dip (S45, page 187)

FLEXIBILITY STRETCHES

LOWER-BODY STRETCHES: LEGS
S1. **Downward Dog**

BENEFIT This outstanding whole-body stretch affects the entire posterior muscle chain and helps strengthen the legs, hips, and shoulders. This pose is a must.

DIRECTIONS Start on the floor on all fours. Raise your hips and straighten your legs. Focus on pushing your knees out through the backs of your legs while pressing your heels toward the floor. At the same time, raise your tailbone to the ceiling. Pressing into the floor with your hands, try to get your body shaped like a V *(Fig. 11.1)* and remember to breathe. Hold this pose for 30 seconds.

Fig. 11.1 Body shaped like a V

S2. **Spread-Foot Forward Bend**

BENEFIT This wonderful stretch for the adductors, inner thighs, hamstrings, and lower back results in a greater rotation of the hips and allows the forward leg to separate from the trailing leg during the forward swing.

DIRECTIONS Spread your feet wide and keep your legs tight while bending forward, placing your hands on the floor *(Fig. 11.2)*. The ideal is to have your fingertips in line with your toes. If that is unattainable, place your hands wherever it is comfortable. If you can't reach the floor without bending your knees, use a prop, such as a yoga block or exercise ball. Breathe deeply for 20 to 30 seconds.

Fig. 11.2 Whether you use a prop or not, keep your legs tight

S3. **Runner's Stretch**

BENEFIT This stretches the hamstrings and calves. Hamstring flexibility contributes to mobilization and stabilization of the hips and helps keep the knees flexed and loaded.

DIRECTIONS You will need a chair for this stretch. Start by kneeling on the floor and put both hands on the top of a chair. Place your

Fig. 11.3 Place both hands on top of chair

Fig. 11.4 Walk your hands down the chair, keeping your front knee straight

right foot forward, pointing straight ahead. Bring your left knee flush up against your right heel. (If you have knee problems and it is difficult for you to get down on the floor, you may start from a standing position, making sure that both feet are in line with each other.) Slowly stand up, straightening both knees, especially your front knee, and make sure your rear foot is flat on the floor *(Fig. 11.3)*.

Begin walking your hands down the chair, attempting to get your fingertips to the floor *(Fig. 11.4)*. However, do not let your front knee bend. When you feel the back of your front knee begin to burn, back off slightly and breathe deeper. It's not how far down to the floor you get that counts, but rather how deeply you breathe into the stretch. You'll notice that, as you breathe, you will drop a little more. Don't force this stretch, but rather breathe into it. Hold for 30 to 60 seconds. Repeat on the other side.

S4. Single-Leg Pelvic Tilt

BENEFIT This active stretch warms up the lower-back muscles and prepares the back for other stretches. In the golf swing, this stretch allows the lower back to flex forward more easily in the stance.

DIRECTIONS Lie on your back with your legs straight. Bend your exercising leg. Place one hand either behind your knee or both hands on your kneecap. Using your abdominals, pull your knee back toward your armpit as you exhale *(Fig. 11.5)*. Hold for 1 to 2 seconds, release, and inhale. Switch and do the other side. Do 5 to 10 repetitions.

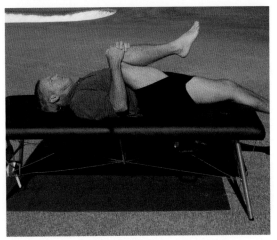

Fig. 11.5 Knee pulled back

S5. Double-Leg Pelvic Tilt

BENEFIT This stretch warms up both sides simultaneously.

DIRECTIONS Lie on your back as directed in the single-leg pelvic tilt (S4). This time, take hold of both knees and pull them back toward your armpits as you exhale *(Fig. 11.6)*. Hold for 1 to 2 seconds, release, and inhale. Do 5 to 10 repetitions.

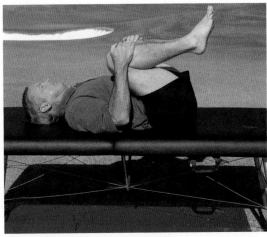

Fig. 11.6 Both knees pulled back

S6. Bent-Knee Hamstring Stretch

BENEFIT This stretches out the lower-hamstring muscle, just above and behind the knee. Keeping the lower hamstring flexible allows the knee and pelvis to remain stable and flexed throughout the golf swing. Inflexible hamstrings make it difficult for any golfer to keep the knees flexed and stay down into the shot. This stretch is a preparatory stretch for the straight-leg hamstring stretch (S8, opposite page).

DIRECTIONS You will need a rope for this stretch. Lie on your back and bend your right knee. Raise your right leg so that your thigh is perpendicular to the floor and your lower leg is parallel to the floor. Place your left hand on your lower right thigh just above your knee to stabilize your leg. Holding a rope in your right hand, place the rope around the bottom of your right foot *(Fig. 11.7)*. Begin exhaling, contract your right quad, and raise your lower leg so that it's pointing toward the ceiling *(Fig. 11.8)*. Make sure your foot is always pulled back. Apply some pressure at the end of the stretch, holding for 1 to 2 seconds. Don't lift your pelvis off the floor and don't force the stretch. If your flexibility won't allow you to get your leg perpendicular to the floor, you may have to lower your thigh slightly in the starting position. Perform 5 to 10 repetitions. Repeat on the other side.

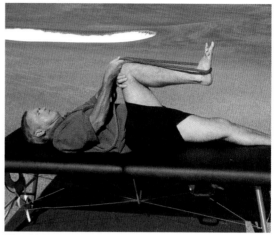

Fig. 11.7 Rope placed around bottom of right foot

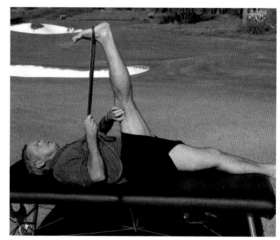

Fig. 11.8 Leg pointing toward ceiling

S7. Supine Leg Chain

BENEFIT This is a great exercise for stretching all of the muscles in the posterior muscle chain, from the glutes on down to your calves.

DIRECTIONS You will need a rope for this stretch. Lie on your back with both of your legs extended. Wrap the rope around the balls of your feet and make sure your feet are pulled back toward you. Gently lift your legs up as far as you can without bending your knees and while keeping your lower back pressed to the floor *(Fig. 11.9)*. As you're pulling your feet and legs toward you with the rope, you should be simultaneously pushing your legs away from you, creating isometric/eccentric contraction.

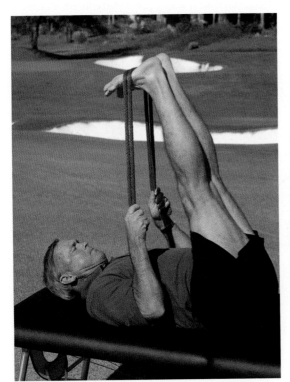

Fig. 11.9 Keep your legs straight and lower back pressed down

S8. Straight-Leg Hamstring Stretch

BENEFIT This stretches out the main belly of the hamstring. A functional hamstring allows for the stability of the pelvis and maintaining flex in the knees throughout the golf swing. Tight hamstrings often result in the straightening of the legs and a loss of mobility and stability during the swing.

DIRECTIONS You will need a rope for this stretch. Lie on your back with your legs straight. Place the rope around the ball of your right foot. Arch your foot back and lift your leg up *(Fig. 11.10)*, always keeping your knees locked. If you feel pressure in your lower back, bend the opposite knee for relief. At the end of the stretch, give a gentle tug on the rope and hold for 1 to 2 seconds. Repeat 5 to 10 times on each side.

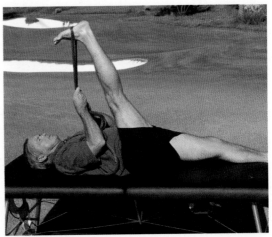

Fig. 11.10 Foot arched with leg up

S9. **Adductor Stretch**

BENEFIT This stretch allows the inner thighs to remain flexible, which will free up the pelvis and allow it to rotate to maximum capacity. This will also allow the left leg to separate from the right on the downswing.

DIRECTIONS You will need a rope for this stretch. Lie on your back with both legs extended and your feet pigeon-toed. Place the rope around

Fig. 11.11 Rope placement

Fig. 11.12 Leg extended to the side

your right foot, then wrap it to the inside of your right leg and then back around to the outside of the leg *(Fig. 11.11)*. Hold the rope with your left hand. Keep your leg straight (and your foot still pigeon-toed), and gently extend your leg out to the side as far as you can without straining *(Fig. 11.12)*. Give a gentle tug to the rope at the end of the stretch and hold for 1 to 2 seconds. Repeat and do the other side. For a full workout, do 5 to 10 repetitions on each side.

S10. **Abductor Stretch**

BENEFIT This exercise stretches the outer thighs and hips, allowing the lower body to stabilize throughout the swing. Tight hips slow down the centrifugal force created during the golf swing.

DIRECTIONS You will need a rope for this stretch. Lie on your back with both legs extended and your feet flared, both facing in the same direction. Both feet should be facing away from the direction you are going to stretch (i.e., if you are stretching your right leg to the left, both feet should face right). Place the rope around your right foot, then wrap it to the outside of your right leg and then back around to the inside of the leg *(Fig. 11.13)*. Hold the rope with your right hand. Keeping your leg relatively straight and the foot flared out, gently extend the leg across your body as far as you can without straining *(Fig. 11.14)*. Use the opposite hand to gently tug on the rope at the end of the stretch and hold for 1 to 2 seconds.

Try not to raise your leg too high. You'll feel this in the outside of the upper thigh. Repeat and do the other side. For a full workout, do 5 to 10 repetitions on each side.

Fig. 11.13 Rope placement

Fig. 11.14 Leg extended across the body

S11. Quadriceps Stretch

BENEFIT This stretch loosens up the quadriceps muscles, which are too tight in most people. This stretch allows the knees, legs, and hips to synchronize and work together.

DIRECTIONS You will need a rope for this stretch. Double loop a rope around your lower right leg. Lie on your side with your thigh in line with your torso. Pull your right foot back to your buttocks and hold for 1 to 2 seconds *(Fig. 11.15)*. Release back to the starting position. Make sure that you don't allow your thigh to go forward of your torso. Repeat 5 to 10 times on each side.

Fig. 11.15 Pull the foot back to the buttocks. Don't allow the thigh to go forward.

Alternate (S11A): Standing Quadriceps Stretch

DIRECTIONS Standing with your thighs in line with your torso, grab your right foot. Bring it up toward your buttocks *(Fig. 11.16)*. Try not to lean forward. Hold for 1 to 2 seconds and

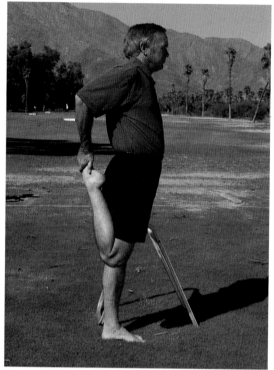

Fig. 11.16 Foot behind buttocks, pressed down

release. This may be done either as an active stretch (5 to 10 times each side), or as a static stretch (20 seconds each side).

LOWER-BODY STRETCHES: HIPS
S12. Standing Drop-Off (with Gluteal Contractions)

BENEFIT This is a powerful pose that helps restore the ankle, knee, hip, and shoulder relationship. In addition, it helps release your hips and at the same time strengthens your glutes and puts them in a neutral position, which will allow your shoulders to come back into proper

position. This pose is a must for people who want to improve their posture.

DIRECTIONS You will need a slant board for this stretch. Stand on a slant board (a plank of wood, a footstool, or another appropriate replacement is fine) against a wall with your heels below your toes *(Fig. 11.17)*. If you use a footstool, stand on the edge—on the balls of your feet, allowing your heels to drop down. Make sure that your heels are against the wall *(Fig. 11.18)*. It is important to have your feet pointing straight ahead and directly in line with your hips and shoulders. Although we want the toes to be angled upward, there should

Fig. 11.17 Stand on a slant board and continually squeeze and release glutes

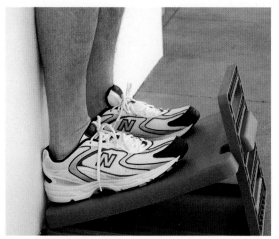

Fig. 11.18 Heels against wall

be no discomfort in the pose. Let your body relax. Now begin to gently but firmly contract (squeeze) your glutes (your fanny). Hold for 1 second and release. Continue to contract them for the entire duration of the exercise.

When you're finished with the pose and you step off the prop, you'll be amazed at the lifting of the upper thorax and the improved posture that you'll suddenly attain.

You can stay in this pose up to 10 minutes for therapy, and eventually cut it down to 2 to 4 minutes. (This pose is one of my personal favorites, and I do it every day.)

S13. **Active Groin Stretch**

BENEFIT This is a great pose that uses gravity to relax and loosen the powerful hip flexors. Relaxing the hips is crucial in developing superb flexibility.

DIRECTIONS Lie on a table, making sure that your tailbone is off the edge and pushing into the end of the table. Clasp your hands and place them under the back of your right knee. Make sure that your right thigh is perpendicular to the table (*Fig. 11.19*). There should be a small arch in your back. Relax your extended (right) leg completely and also relax your upper body. Hold for 1 minute and switch to the other leg. You'll notice that your extended leg will begin to relax completely. If you want to stay in the stretch longer, by all means do so.

Fig. 11.19 Lie at the end of a table and relax hips and shoulders

S14. **Psoas Stretch**

BENEFIT This stretch is a must for the hips.

DIRECTIONS Kneel on the floor with your feet, knees, hips, and shoulders approximately in a straight line. Place your forward foot approximately 18 to 24 inches in front of your back knee. Keep your spine vertical and sink down toward the floor as you lift your chest *(Fig. 11.20)*. You should feel this deep in your groin. If your stability is good, you can raise your arms over your head or even place a golf club behind your back for increased extension. Hold this pose for 20 to 30 seconds on static stretches and do 5 to 10 repetitions for active stretches. Switch and do the other side.

Fig. 11.20 Kneeling psoas stretch

Alternate (S14A): Standing Psoas Stretch

I recommend that most people do this stretch in a standing position several times a day to counter the effects of our sedentary lifestyle *(Fig. 11.21)*.

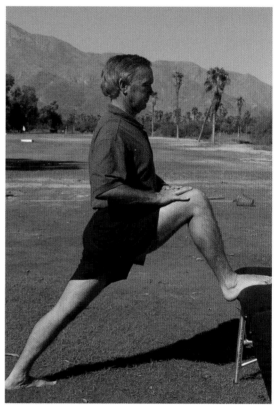

Fig. 11.21 Standing psoas stretch

S15. **Warrior II**

BENEFIT This pose develops strength and flexibility in the legs and also brings elasticity to the back muscles.

DIRECTIONS Stand at attention. Spread your feet approximately 4 feet apart, keeping your right foot straight ahead and turning your left foot outward 90 degrees. The ankles should be in a direct line with one another. Exhale and bend your left knee so that your thigh is parallel to the floor. (If you can't go down that low, don't worry about it—just do the best you can.) The bent knee should be in line with the ankle, and not extending beyond it. Keep your right leg straight. Stretch out your arms and hands sideways as though two people are pulling you from each end *(Fig. 11.22)*. Your chest should be facing the direction that you started. Turn your head so you are looking out over your extended left arm. Hold for 20 to 30 seconds. Switch and do the other side.

Fig. 11.22 Keep your torso as straight as possible

S16. **Sitting Wall**

BENEFIT This great hamstrings and glutes stretch sets the pelvis, which aids in attaining better posture and stabilizing the hips in the address position, as well as maintaining a proper spine angle throughout the swing.

DIRECTIONS Sit against a wall at attention. Press your shoulders into the wall and make sure that your tailbone is as close to the wall as possible. In the beginning, if it's too uncomfortable to get your tailbone close to the wall, back off until it's manageable. In time this will become easier to do. As you press your shoulders back, be sure to lift your sternum as you breathe deeply and fully with your abdomen, making sure you push your abdomen outward on the inhalation. Pull your feet back while pressing your knees to the floor *(Fig. 11.23)*. Try to keep your chin level and your head against the wall. Many people won't be able to get their head back against the wall while keeping their chin level, but do the best you can. This pose is very difficult for many people, so don't force it. Pay attention and breathe. Hold for 1 to 2 minutes. For a more advanced pose, try to keep your heels off the floor.

Fig. 11.23 Legs straight, feet arched back

S17. Solo Sitting Wall

BENEFIT This powerful pose not only stretches the hamstrings but also helps lengthen the anterior muscle chain (the iliacus, psoas, and diaphragm), whose dysfunction is epidemic in our digital world. The benefits of this pose extend far beyond the musculoskeletal world and will help create better health and fitness because of the improved function of the diaphragm.

DIRECTIONS You will need a half-round foam roller (or a towel) and a rope for this stretch. Sit against a wall at attention. Take the foam roller (or a towel rolled to 6 to 8 inches in diameter), and place it behind your back near the bottom of your shoulder blades *(Fig. 11.24)*. Press your shoulders into the foam roller as if you were trying to get your shoulders to touch the wall. At the same time try to get the back of your head to touch the wall, but don't let your head arch backward. Keep your jawline level, even if you can't get your head to touch the wall. Breathe deeply while lifting your sternum and expanding your abdomen.

For a more advanced stretch, wrap a rope around the soles of your feet and pull your feet back toward you while pushing your knees to the floor *(Fig. 11.25)*. For many people, this is very uncomfortable in the beginning, so be sure not to force the pose.

The primary focus should be on pressing your shoulders back toward the wall and breathing deeply. The secondary focus should be on pulling your feet back and your knees toward the floor. Many people bend forward while they pull their feet back, which is counterproductive. Hold this pose for 2 to 4 minutes in the beginning. As you get more proficient, cut down the time to 1 to 2 minutes.

Fig. 11.24 Half-round foam roller behind shoulder blades

Fig. 11.25 Use a rope to pull back feet

S18. **Hip-Thigh Extension**

In addition to flexibility, we must also have a good balance of strength in the muscle groups, which will allow the body to achieve stability. This is especially true in the posterior muscles, particularly the glutes. Due to the forward-bending flexion culture we live in, the muscles of our anterior (front muscles) get too tight and pull the torso forward, thus weakening and tightening the posterior (rear muscles). As a result, our back muscles generally become weaker, thus preventing the necessary stability that is so crucial for our golf swings.

BENEFIT These extensions are terrific for strengthening back-side muscles while stretching the front side.

DIRECTIONS Lying supine on the floor, bend your left knee and straighten your right leg *(Fig. 11.26)*. Your palms should be faceup about 45 degrees from your body. Now lift your entire body up 1 to 2 inches by pushing off your left foot *(Fig. 11.27)*. This is the start position. Continue to lift your entire body in a straight line so that your thighs are parallel to each other *(Fig. 11.28)*. The only parts of your body that are in contact with the floor are your arms, upper back, and left foot. Remember that when you lift, you're lifting primarily with your torso, not just your leg. The extended leg just goes along for the ride.

Hold for 3 seconds and lower yourself back down to 1 inch off the floor. Pause and repeat 5 to 10 times. Be sure to keep your hips in a straight line. Repeat on the other side and eventually build up your repetitions.

Fig. 11.26 Left knee bent with straight right leg

Fig. 11.27 Lift with your torso, not just your leg

Fig. 11.28 Body in a straight line with thighs parallel

S19. Hip Crossover

BENEFIT This is an excellent exercise for creating bilateral mobility in both hips, which also aids in developing a greater shoulder turn.

DIRECTIONS Lie on the floor with both knees bent, your feet flat on the floor and your arms out to your sides. Raise your left leg so that your left thigh is perpendicular to the floor and your lower left leg is parallel to the floor. Cross your right ankle over your left knee and slightly press your right knee away from you *(Fig. 11.29)*. Now roll your right knee and foot over to the left so that your right foot is firmly on the floor *(Fig. 11.30)*. Don't force this stretch. As you roll over, make sure that you apply slight pressure on the knee (pushing it forward), while you look in the opposite direction with your head. Hold this pose for 1 minute. Switch and do the other side.

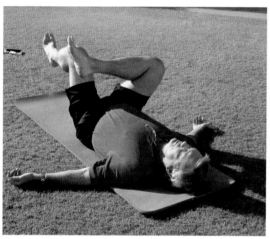

Fig. 11.29 Right ankle over left knee

Fig. 11.30 Right knee and right foot over left, firmly on floor

S20. **Internal and External Hip Rotators**

`BENEFIT` This stretch helps open the powerful deep-six rotators in the hips, which allow the lateral rotation of the thighs. This will allow the hips to turn in an unrestricted manner in the golf swing.

`DIRECTIONS` You will need a rope for this stretch. Lie on your back with your knees bent. Bend your right knee and place the rope under your right foot and wrap it to the inside of your lower leg and then back to the outside. Hold the rope in your right hand. Your thigh should be 90 degrees to the floor and 90 degrees to your lower leg *(Fig. 11.31)*. Place your left hand on your right thigh just above the knee for stability. Now slowly rotate your calf and foot outward *(Fig. 11.32)*, making sure that your right thigh remains perpendicular to the floor. Hold for 1 to 2 seconds. Repeat 5 to 10 times.

After finishing the outward movements, turn your lower calf inward *(Fig. 11.33)* and repeat 5 to 10 times. When your leg goes inward (internal rotation), hold the rope with the opposite hand. When your leg goes outward (external rotation), hold the rope with the same-side hand. Repeat with the other leg.

Fig. 11.31 Thigh is perpendicular to the floor and lower leg 90 degrees to the thigh

Fig. 11.32 Rotate calf outward

Fig. 11.33 Rotate calf inward

Fig. 11.34 Soles of feet together with knees turned out

S21. **Frog**

BENEFIT This stretch allows your inner thighs to stretch and helps release the hips, relaxing the adductors and helping free up the pelvis.

DIRECTIONS Place your arms at a 45-degree angle with the backs of your hands on the floor. Lie on your back and bring your feet up toward your torso. Bring the soles of your feet together, allowing your knees to turn out *(Fig. 11.34)*. Do not force your knees down, but allow your thighs to gently relax into a comfortable position. Hold for 1 to 2 minutes.

Alternate (S21A): Elevated Frog (Advanced)

BENEFIT This is a more advanced stretch that helps strengthen the glutes as you stretch your hip flexors. This also helps tame the nerves in the sympathetic nervous system located in your solar plexus.

DIRECTIONS Lift your pelvis well off the floor, making sure to keep your knees open and relaxed *(Fig. 11.35)*. It doesn't matter where you place your arms. They can be above your head, next to your body, or on your belly. Simply find the most comfortable position for them. Hold for 1 to 2 minutes.

Fig. 11.35 Lift pelvis off the floor, keeping knees open

LOWER BODY AND UPPER TRUNK
S22. Counter

BENEFIT This stretches the hamstrings, glutes, and shoulders, allowing you to stabilize and maintain a proper hip tilt throughout the swing.

DIRECTIONS From the overhead extension (S35, page 176) and facing a wall, lean forward and place your hands against the wall so that your arms and upper torso are 90 degrees to your lower body. Keeping your weight on the balls of your feet, push your hands into the wall, extending your torso with your legs tight *(Fig. 11.36)*. Hold for 20 seconds.

Fig. 11.36 Push your hands into the wall, extending your torso

S23. Cats and Dogs

BENEFIT This excellent stretch for the hips, back, chest, and spine helps the hips and shoulders work together and increases range of motion of the pelvis and spine throughout the swing.

DIRECTIONS Start on the floor in an all-fours position with your hands under your shoulders and your knees under your hips. Breathe out as you arch your back up (like a scared cat) while looking at your navel *(Fig. 11.37)*. Then breathe in as you slowly arch your back down while looking up at the ceiling (like a happy dog *[Fig. 11.38]*). Don't rock back and forth. Hold each position for 1 to 2 seconds. Repeat 5 to 8 times.

Fig. 11.37 Arched back (cat)

Fig. 11.38 Back down (dog)

S24. **Bridge**

BENEFIT This stretches the abdominals and hip flexors and strengthens the glutes and lower back. It increases range of motion in the trunk and adds stability and power to the swing.

DIRECTIONS Lie on your back with your knees bent and your arms at your sides. Gently raise your hips *(Fig. 11.39)* and hold for 20 seconds.

Fig. 11.39 Hips raised

S25. **Cobra**

BENEFIT This is an excellent stretch for the torso.

DIRECTIONS Lie facedown on the floor with both forearms resting on the floor, slightly in front of your shoulders. Gently straighten your arms *(Fig. 11.40)*, lifting your head and sternum up higher. Go easy here because this puts a lot of friction on your lower back. Relax your buttocks as you look up toward the ceiling. Hold for 5 seconds.

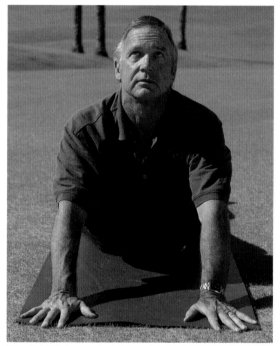

Fig. 11.40 Arms straightened

S26. Triangle

BENEFIT This exercise works a multitude of the body's muscle groups at the same time. In addition to stretching the hamstrings, hips, chest, and lower back, the triangle also stretches out the lats and obliques (on your sides), which allow the body to achieve a maximum torso turn and create arm extension. This is also great for helping to eliminate the chicken wing.

DIRECTIONS Stand with your back against a wall and your feet slightly wider than shoulder width. Flare your right foot approximately 90 degrees in the direction you're going to lean. If you have bad knees, keep your feet pointing straight ahead. Flare your arms and hands directly out to your sides with your shoulders firmly against the wall *(Fig. 11.41)*. Keep the backs of your hands, arms, and shoulders against the wall at all times. Slowly drop your lead arm down as far as you can without forcing it. Make sure your shoulders and arms stay pressed to the wall. Slowly look up at the top arm, making sure it too is against the wall *(Fig. 11.42)*. You'll feel this stretch in your lats (side muscles). Breathe deeply and fully, expanding your ribs, and relax. Hold for 20 to 30 seconds on each side. It's not how far down you go that counts, but how deeply you breathe while maintaining the integrity of your posture.

Fig. 11.41 Press your hands, arms, shoulders, and hips against the wall

Fig. 11.42 One arm dropped down with both arms against the wall

S27. **Extended Lateral**

BENEFIT This pose is excellent for developing function (mobility and stability) in your legs as well as creating bilateral hip activity on both sides of your torso. Like the triangle (S26, page 167), it increases range of motion in the muscles of your sides (lats and obliques), as well as developing strength in your legs, which will help create greater ease in trunk rotation and synchronize all of your body's major muscle groups.

DIRECTIONS Stand with your back against a wall and your arms extended and heels and buttocks touching the wall. Take your right foot, turn it parallel to the wall, and spread your feet about 3 to 4 feet apart, bending your right knee slightly but keeping your left leg straight *(Fig. 11.43)*. Your right foot should be 3 inches from the wall. Lean your entire upper torso toward your right foot. Place your right arm on your right thigh. Raise your left arm over your head and look up toward the ceiling *(Fig. 11.44)*. Make sure that your shoulders and hips stay pressed against the wall. Hold for 20 to 30 seconds. Repeat on the other side.

Fig. 11.43 Starting position

Fig. 11.44 Ending position

S28. The Bow

BENEFIT This pose complements the solo sitting wall (S17, page 160) by further stretching out the anterior muscles and contracting the posterior muscles.

DIRECTIONS Lie facedown on the floor. Bend your knees and feet back toward your head. Grab each ankle with your hands and arch backward *(Fig. 11.45)*. Hold the pose for 20 seconds.

Many people will not be able to grab their ankles. If you can't, use a rope or stretch bands for assistance, or use the alternate extended half bow (S28A).

Alternate (S28A): Extended Half Bow

BENEFIT This is an excellent stretch that provides strengthening, flexibility, and extension to the core muscle group.

DIRECTIONS Lie facedown on the floor. Take your right hand and grab your right ankle and simultaneously extend your left arm forward *(Fig. 11.46)*. Now gently lift your right leg off the floor while you gently pull the right foot toward your head. At the same time, extend with your left arm while you're lifting your chest off the floor. Hold for 15 to 20 seconds. Repeat on the other side.

Fig. 11.45 Hands holding ankles, arched backward

Fig. 11.46 Right hand grabs right ankle and left arm extends forward

S29. **Seated Forward Bend**

BENEFIT This stretch warms up the muscles of the spine to prepare for the spinal twists that follow. Warming up the erector spinae muscles is important in allowing the spine to rotate during the golf swing.

DIRECTIONS Sit on the edge of a chair with your back straight *(Fig. 11.47)*. Tuck your chin down and grasp the sides of your legs or the legs of the chair as you pull your body forward *(Fig. 11.48)*. Hold for 1 to 2 seconds and come up. Breathe deeply and fully. Repeat 5 to 10 times.

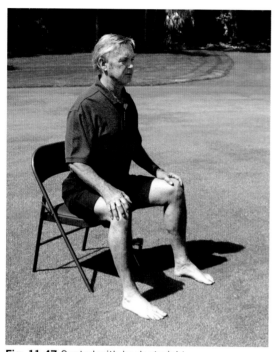

Fig. 11.47 Seated with back straight

Fig. 11.48 Grasping legs and pulling body forward

S30. **Oblique Side Flex**

WARNING Do not do this stretch if you have disc or back problems.

BENEFIT Want a better shoulder turn? This exercise stretches your obliques, which will increase your trunk rotation on both sides of the ball.

DIRECTIONS Sit on the edge of a chair in an upright position. Clasp your hands and place them behind your head *(Fig. 11.49)*. Maintaining your posture, inhale and gently twist to the left side *(Fig. 11.50)*. Exhaling, lead with your right elbow and sink down toward the floor *(Fig. 11.51)*. Try to keep your left elbow pointing up and behind you. Do not force this, but maintain your posture. Hold for 2 seconds and inhale as you return to the starting position. Think "Upright posture, rotate, down." Do 5 to 10 repetitions, repeat on the other side.

Fig. 11.49 Seated with back straight

Fig. 11.50 Gently twist to one side

Fig. 11.51 Sink down toward floor

SPINAL TWISTS

`WARNING` Use care or don't perform the following back exercises if you have back problems or have been injured.

S31. Pretzel

`BENEFIT` A stretch for the lower lumbar and obliques, this aids in developing a greater shoulder turn.

`DIRECTIONS` Sit on the floor with your legs extended and your back as straight as possible. Place your right foot just outside your left knee, making sure you keep the foot flat on the floor. Initially, it doesn't matter how far up your leg you place your foot. Now take your right hand and place it directly behind the midline of your body. With your left arm straight, press it against your right thigh, just above your knee. Lift your sternum and look as far behind you as you can. Breathe deeply while pressing your left arm against your right thigh *(Fig. 11.52)*. Hold the pose for 30 to 45 seconds. Repeat on the other side.

Alternate (S31A): Pretzel in Chair

An easier way to do the pretzel is in a chair. Sit sideways on a chair (with the backrest to your side). Place both hands on the top of the backrest. With your feet solidly on the floor, twist your torso rearward while looking behind you as far as you can *(Fig. 11.53)*. Hold for the desired time or repetitions.

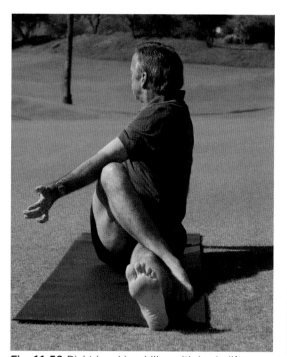

Fig. 11.52 Right hand is midline with back; lift sternum

Fig. 11.53 Alternate pretzel stretch

S32. **Upper Spinal Floor Twist**

BENEFIT The upper spine rotates approximately 60 to 70 percent more than the lower spine in the golf swing. When a person has rounded shoulders, this tightness inhibits the freedom of the shoulder turn. This pose stretches out and relaxes the anterior muscles in the upper chest and shoulders.

DIRECTIONS Lie on one side in a fetal position with your calves, thighs, torso, and arms at a 90-degree angle. Keep your knees pressed against a prop *(Fig. 11.54)*. Place your arms straight out in front of you with your hands together, as if in prayer *(Fig. 11.55)*. Take your top hand and arm and slowly swing them all the way over to the other side toward the floor *(Fig. 11.56)*. Keep the bottom hand on the floor and make sure that you keep your knees pressed against the prop. Relax and notice that your extended hand, arm, and shoulder will begin to enter into deeper levels of relaxation, slowly getting closer to the floor. If your shoulders get sore, simply lower the arm closer to your torso to ease the torque. Hold for 1 minute. Repeat on the other side.

Fig. 11.54 Keep your knees pressed against a prop

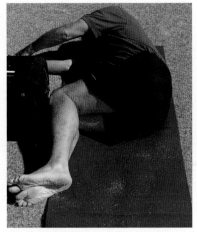

Fig. 11.55 Arms straight out with hands together

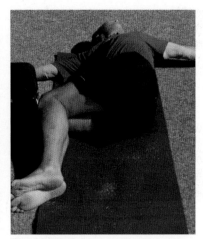

Fig. 11.56 Swing your top arm over, keeping your knees against the prop

S33. **Crocodile**

BENEFIT Another great stretch for increasing your shoulder turn, this pose stretches the muscles of the spine as well as the obliques and also helps achieve maximum rotation of the thorax.

DIRECTIONS Lie on your back with your legs extended and your feet pointed straight up. Put the heel of your right foot on top of the toes of your left foot. Extend your arms out to your sides with your palms facing down *(Fig. 11.57)*. Keeping your legs tight and your feet arched back toward you, roll your hips and legs over to the left while pressing into the floor with your hands. The success of this pose depends on keeping your legs tight and your feet arched back. Don't worry if you can't get your feet to touch the floor. Turn your head to the right, countering the force of your hips *(Fig. 11.58)*. Hold this position for 1 minute. Repeat on the other side.

Fig. 11.57 Arms out and palms facing down

Fig. 11.58 Turn the head to the opposite side that your body is twisting.

S34. **Russian Ball Twist**

BENEFIT These twists will increase your core strength and improve your trunk rotation.

DIRECTIONS You will need an exercise ball for this stretch. Place your back, shoulders, and head on the ball. Lift your hips up so that they're in a straight line with your torso. Holding your arms straight up in front of you (perpendicular to the floor), clasp your hands together. Place your tongue on the roof of your mouth to allow greater oxygenation. Begin rotating your trunk as far as possible from side to side, using a slow and deliberate tempo *(Figs. 11.59 and 11.60)*. Hold for 2 seconds on each side at the end of the exercise. Make sure to keep your hips up at all times.

MODERATE WORKOUT Perform 5 to 10 repetitions.

ADVANCED WORKOUT Increase repetitions or do two to three sets of 5 to 10 repetitions.

Fig. 11.59 Rotate your trunk onto your shoulder

Fig. 11.60 Rotate to the other side

SHOULDERS
S35. Overhead Extension

BENEFIT This is an excellent opening warmup stretch that oxygenates the entire body and prepares the muscles for the remainder of the program.

DIRECTIONS Stand at attention (preferably against a wall). Keep your legs tight and raise your arms as high as they'll go while keeping your shoulder blades pressed together *(Fig. 11.61)*. Push your pelvis slightly forward. Don't force this stretch, and remember to breathe. Hold for 10 seconds.

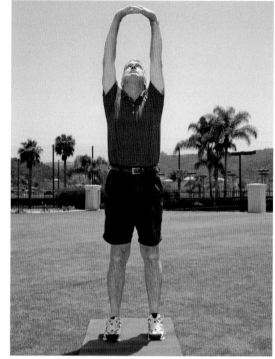

Fig 11.61 Arms high

S36. **Pectorals (Pecs) Stretch**

BENEFIT This exercise stretches out the muscles of the chest and shoulders, which tend to shorten due to our forward-flexion culture. Stretching the anterior muscles of the shoulders allows you to expand the muscles on the backswing, making a freer and fuller shoulder turn.

DIRECTIONS Pec stretches can be done a number of ways. Standing with your feet shoulder-width apart, place your arms at eight o'clock and four o'clock and stretch them rearward *(Fig. 11.62)*, holding for 1 to 2 seconds. Move your arms to nine o'clock and three o'clock and hold for 1 to 2 seconds *(Fig. 11.63)*. Then move your arms up to ten o'clock and two o'clock *(Fig. 11.64)* and hold for 1 to 2 seconds. Repeat each position 3 times.

Fig. 11.62 Arms at eight o'clock and four o'clock

Fig. 11.63 Arms at nine o'clock and three o'clock

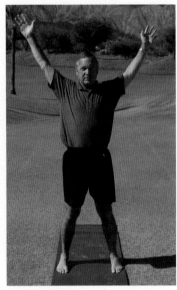

Fig. 11.64 Arms at ten o'clock and two o'clock

Alternate (S36A): Pec in Doorway

Another way to do the pectorals stretch is to use a doorway *(Fig. 11.65)* and allow your body weight to lean forward.

Fig. 11.65 In a doorway

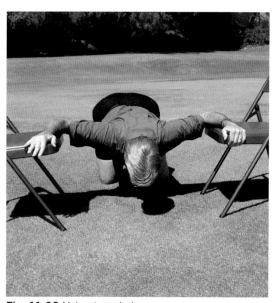

Fig. 11.66 Using two chairs as props

Alternate (S36B): Pec with Chairs

Still another method is to use two chairs, or other props.

DIRECTIONS Get down on your knees and place your forearms on each chair so that your knees are directly underneath your hips and your arms are 90 degrees from your torso *(Fig. 11.66)*. Gently lower your torso so you feel the stretch in your chest and shoulder blades. Don't force it, but rather concentrate on your breathing.

S37. Arm Circle

BENEFIT This stretch strengthens the muscles of the back while increasing range of motion in the shoulder sockets and creating greater freedom of the arms throughout the golf swing.

DIRECTIONS Stand upright with your chest lifted and your feet squared. With your arms hanging at your sides, place your hands with your fingertips curled inward and your thumbs outward *(Fig. 11.67)*. We call this the "golfer's grip." Raise your arms out to your sides at shoulder level, parallel to the floor, with your

Fig. 11.67 Golfer's grip

Fig. **11.68** Arms at shoulder level

Fig. **11.69** Palms facing ceiling

palms facedown *(Fig. 11.68)*. Keeping your shoulder blades pressed together, rotate your arms in approximately 6-inch-diameter circles, gradually increasing the size of the circles. After approximately 40 circles, turn your hands palms up to face the ceiling and do 40 more repetitions *(Fig. 11.69)*, then circling backward.

You can increase this number as you see fit. Keep your shoulders back and your chest lifted at all times.

S38. **Elbow Curl**

BENEFIT This stretch engages the posterior muscles of the upper back, enhancing range of motion in the shoulder sockets and creating greater freedom of the arms throughout the golf swing.

DIRECTIONS Stand upright and, using the golfer's grip *(Fig. 11.67)*, place your knuckles against your temples with your upper arms parallel to the floor and your thumbs facing down. Keeping your arms parallel to the floor, bring your elbows in toward each other until they touch *(Fig. 11.70)*. (If they can't touch, then you have excessive tightness in your upper chest and shoulders.) Hold this position for 1 second and then extend your elbows behind you as far as they will go—without straining—and hold for 1 second *(Fig. 11.71)*. Repeat 10 to 20 times.

Fig. 11.70 Knuckles against temples and elbows touching

Fig. 11.71 Elbows extended to maximum position

S39. **Why Me**

BENEFIT This stretch increases range of motion in the pecs and shoulders.

DIRECTIONS Stand with your arms parallel to the floor, with your hands facing each other—fingers pointing to the floor and palms facing outward (11.72). Raise your arms while simultaneously rotating your arms and palms inward. Your upper and lower arms should resemble a goalpost *(Fig. 11.73)*. Hold for 2 seconds at the top of the movement and repeat 8 to 10 times.

Fig. 11.72 Palms facing outward

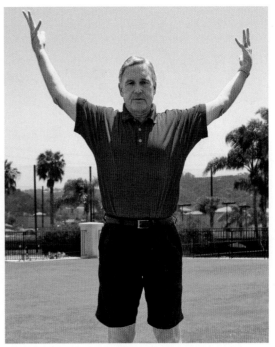

Fig. 11.73 Forearms rotated, palms facing each other

S40. **Breaststroke**

BENEFIT This stretch increases range of motion in the pecs and shoulders.

DIRECTIONS Place your forearms parallel to the floor, hands together, with your fingers extended and pointing toward your chest *(Fig. 11.74)*. Roll your thumbs in toward your chest, and then extend your arms out as if you were doing a breaststroke in the pool *(Fig. 11.75)*. Repeat 8 to 10 times.

Fig. 11.74 Forearms parallel to the floor, fingers pointing toward chest

Fig. 11.75 Arms extended

S41. **Lateral Ball Roll**

BENEFIT This stretch is powerful and improves many areas of the body at the same time, especially the posterior muscles of your back and shoulders.

DIRECTIONS You will need an exercise ball for this stretch. Position your body so that your head and the area between your shoulder blades are comfortably supported on the ball. Lift your hips so that they are in a straight line with your torso. Extend both arms out to the sides and keep your tongue on the roof of your mouth. Begin to roll laterally to one side of the ball, keeping the alignment of your arms parallel to the floor *(Fig. 11.76)*. Start out slowly, eventually shuffling your feet to accommodate going farther out on the edge of the ball *(Fig. 11.77)*. As you progress with this exercise, you'll be able to support yourself with only one shoulder on the ball. Go slowly in the beginning until you build up to that point. As you roll to each side, hold the position for 3 seconds before rolling back to the other side.

Begin by doing 5 to 7 repetitions. Always warm up before doing this exercise. Slowly increase your repetitions as the exercise gets easier to do.

Fig. 11.76 Keep hips in a straight line with torso

Fig. 11.77 Roll from side to side, keeping your arms parallel to the floor and hips elevated

S42. **Internal and External Shoulder Rotators**

BENEFIT These stretches are for achieving more range of motion in the shoulder area, particularly in the rotator cuffs. These stretches will benefit people with tight or rounded shoulders. Loosening these muscles will help you achieve much greater freedom in your shoulder rotation.

Internal Rotators

DIRECTIONS Stand upright with your chest lifted and your shoulders back. Raise your arms out to the sides so that your elbows are level with your shoulders and your palms and forearms are facing the floor *(Fig. 11.78)*. Your arms

should be bent at 90-degree angles to your torso and parallel to the floor. Hold and lock the angle of your elbows as you rotate your arms up. Your lower arms should now be perpendicular to the floor with your palms facing forward *(Fig. 11.79)*. Hold for 2 seconds and return to the starting position and repeat. For maximum stretch, do 8 to 10 repetitions.

External Rotators

DIRECTIONS Begin in the same starting position as the internal rotators *(Fig. 11.78)*. This time, rotate your arms downward *(Fig. 11.80)*. Hold for 2 seconds and return to the starting position and repeat. For a maximum stretch, do 8 to 10 repetitions.

Fig. 11.78 Place hands and arms parallel to the floor

Fig. 11.79 Rotate forearms upward

Fig. 11.80 Arms downward

S43. **Head and Neck Stretches**

WARNING Don't do neck stretches until you've loosened up your hips and upper torso first.

BENEFIT These stretches allow maximum mobility of the upper back and neck. In the golf swing, flexibility in these muscles aids in allowing a free rotation of the cervical spine.

DIRECTIONS Lie on your back on a table or bed with the tops of your shoulders and your head hanging over the edge *(Fig. 11.81)*. Hold this position for 30 seconds to 1 minute. Then tilt your head all the way to the right for 15 seconds. Then tilt your head all the way to the left for 15 seconds *(Fig. 11.82)*. Turn and lie on one side with the top of your shoulder and head hanging over the edge. Look straight down for 15 seconds *(Fig. 11.83)*. Turn and do the same on the other side for 15 seconds. Lastly, sit upright on the edge of the table or bed and tuck your chin down into your sternum for 15 seconds *(Fig. 11.84)*.

Fig. 11.82 Head tilted to the left

Fig. 11.83 Turned onto side and looking down

Fig. 11.81 Head hanging over edge of table in starting position

Fig. 11.84 Sitting upright with chin down

RESISTANCE EXERCISES
S44. Plank

Fig. 11.85 Maintain a straight torso

BENEFIT This core-strengthening exercise develops strength throughout the entire torso. Having a strong core develops stability that goes hand in hand with the flexibility provided in the rest of the program.

DIRECTIONS Lie on your forearms as if you were about to do a pushup, only on your forearms, with your entire body off the floor. Try to keep your hips level with your entire torso *(Fig. 11.85)*. Make sure your breaths are even on the inhales and exhales. After approximately 10 to 15 seconds, raise one leg while keeping your body propped up *(Fig. 11.86)*. Hold for up to 1 minute. Then switch and do the same with the other leg.

Fig. 11.86 Plank with leg extension

Alternate (S44A): Side Plank

DIRECTIONS For a more advanced version of the plank, lie on your side, propped up on your forearm and elbow with the other arm resting alongside your body and your feet stacked on top of each other *(Fig. 11.87)*. Pike your body up, keeping it in a straight line. Make sure you're keeping your shoulder blades close together. Build up to 30 to 60 seconds. Repeat on the other side.

Fig. 11.87 Prop your body on your forearm, keeping your entire torso straight

S45. **Triceps Dip**

BENEFIT This exercise strengthens the triceps and the posterior muscle chains and helps achieve balance between the front and back sides of the torso.

DIRECTIONS Find a chair with a firm armrest, a countertop, or some other firm prop off the floor. Place the palms of your hands on the armrest with your body facing upward and your feet solidly on the floor. Slowly lower your hips to sink toward the floor *(Fig. 11.88)*. Slowly push your palms into the armrests while simultaneously lifting and thrusting your hips upward. Build up to 10 to 20 repetitions.

Note: Don't force this exercise. If you can't go all the way down, it's okay. Simply go easy and build up.

Fig. 11.88 Hands securely on the prop, lowering yourself to tolerance

S46. Baby Dolphin

BENEFIT This stretch strengthens and promotes lumbar and thoracic extension through bilateral hip demand.

DIRECTIONS Start on the floor on all fours with your hip joints above your knees and your shoulders above your wrists. Walk your hands out approximately 6 to 8 inches and then lower your forearms on the floor. Make a fist and slightly rotate your arms so that your thumbs are facing upward *(Fig. 11.89)*. Gently make an arch in your back and gently squeeze your shoulder blades together. You will feel the weight on your forearms and shoulders. Remember to keep squeezing your shoulder blades together. (You may do this pose with your knees elevated on a yoga block, chair, and so forth, if it's not too strenuous for you.) Hold this pose for 30 to 60 seconds.

S47. Dolphin

BENEFIT This pose not only gives a great stretch to your calves and hamstrings but also opens the shoulders and chest and strengthens the arms.

DIRECTIONS Start on the floor on all fours with your hip joints above your knees and your shoulders above your wrists. Now place your elbows where your hands are and either place your palms flat on the floor or make a fist and rotate your forearms so that your thumbs are facing upward.

Curl your toes under and slowly begin to pike your hips upward while straightening your legs. Make sure your knees are tight and that you're constantly pushing your knees back and always pushing your heels to the floor *(Fig. 11.90)*. While you're in the maximum position, be attentive and *gently* squeeze your shoulder blades together. Hold this pose for 30 to 60 seconds.

Fig. 11.89 Majority of weight on forearms

Fig. 11.90 This is a great pose that develops strength and flexibility in the upper and posterior torso.

S48. **Hand-Leg Opposite Lift**

BENEFIT This exercise is tremendous for strengthening and developing greater extension of the spine, pelvis, and hips.

DIRECTIONS Lie on your stomach with one arm stretched overhead and the other down at your side. The arm that is at your side should have the back of the hand on the floor and be pressed against your body. Pigeon-toe your feet with the tops of your feet on the floor. Simultaneously lift the extended arm and the opposite leg off the floor (that is, when you're lifting your right arm, you'll simultaneously be lifting your left leg). Let your head come up with the movement. Hold for a count of 5. Repeat on the other side. Do up to 10 repetitions on each side. This is an excellent workout, but go at your own pace.

Fig. 11.91 Hand-leg opposite lifts ensure strengthening of the posterior erectors and balance the entire body.

S49. **Wall Squat**

BENEFIT This stretch will help you achieve superb lower-body stability in your golf swing by strengthening your legs and hips.

DIRECTIONS You will need an exercise ball for this stretch. Stand with your back against the ball, supported by a wall. Keep your feet, knees, hips, and shoulders in line, making sure your feet are straight ahead *(Fig. 11.92)*. Inhale, then squat down as you exhale *(Fig. 11.93)*. Only go as low as comfortable. Don't let your knees go past your toes and don't let your knees go outside or inside your feet. Stand up, inhaling on the way up. If you have soreness in your knees, be very careful and don't put too much pressure on them. Do 1 to 10 repetitions. Build up the repetitions over time.

Fig. 11.92 Back against ball with feet straight ahead

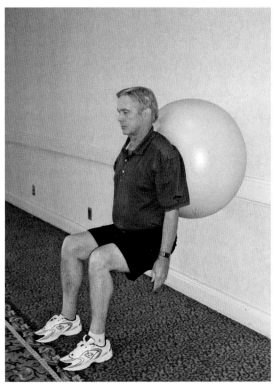

Fig. 11.93 Squat down then back up

S50. Locust

BENEFIT This pose develops a strong and elastic spine and is especially good for people with weak and tight backs.

DIRECTIONS Lie fully extended facedown on the floor. Stretch your arms back with your palms facing up. Exhale and lift your head, chest, and legs off the floor simultaneously *(Fig. 11.94)*. Contract your buttocks and stretch your thigh muscles. Keep both legs fully extended and your arms and feet off the floor. Stay in this position as long as possible while breathing deeply and fully.

Fig. 11.94 Exhale as you lift your head, chest, and legs

Alternate (S50A): Advanced Locust

Clasp your hands around the back of your head *(Fig. 11.95)* and follow the instructions for locust.

Alternate (S50B): Extended Locust

Fig. 11.95 Hands behind head for advanced stretch

BENEFIT This pose develops a strong and elastic spine and is especially good for people with weak and tight backs.

DIRECTIONS You will need stretch bands for this stretch. Place the stretch bands under your feet and hold the other ends in your hands. Elongate your torso as much as possible while you lift your legs, chest, and arms off the floor *(Fig. 11.96)*. Hold for 20 seconds.

Fig. 11.96 Using stretch bands for an advanced stretch

S51. **Air Bench**

`BENEFIT` This exercise strengthens your legs, which will help stabilize your lower body as well as help tame the powerful hip flexors.

`DIRECTIONS` Sit against a wall with the small of your back pressing against the wall. Keep your thighs slightly above parallel to the floor at about a 100- to 110-degree angle *(Fig. 11.97)*. Your knees should be directly above your heels. Make sure that your shoulders, hips, knees, and feet are in alignment, with your feet pointing straight ahead. If this is hard on your knees, modify the pose by squatting a bit less to relieve the pressure. Stay in this pose for 2 minutes.

S52. **Powerful Air Bench**

`BENEFIT` This exercise strengthens the lower body and creates extension through the upper torso.

`DIRECTIONS` Stand in front of a chair. Now press your palms and the forefingers of each hand together. Slowly lower yourself down as if you're about to sit on the chair—only stop a few inches above it *(Fig. 11.98)*. Hold the pose for 2 to 3 seconds and rise back up. Build to tolerance, but try to build up to one set of 10 then eventually two sets of 10.

Fig. 11.97 Thighs slightly above parallel to the floor

Fig. 11.98 Keep arms and back straight while gently squatting downward

RELAXATION POSES

S53. Static Back Press

BENEFIT This pose is extremely important because not only does it relax all the muscles throughout your body, especially the powerful hip flexors, it also helps realign the joints of the body and restore its natural four-socket position.

DIRECTIONS Lie on your back with your knees up on a chair or block *(Fig. 11.99)*. Keep your hands under your shoulders and simply relax for 5 minutes longer. Make sure you breathe deeply by allowing the abdomen to expand outward as you inhale and back inward as you exhale.

Fig. 11.99 Breathe deeply and relax

S54. Supine Groin Stretch

BENEFIT This stretch is very powerful for relaxing and lengthening the hip flexors. Our hips take a beating in our sitting-down culture, and as a result cause a multitude of health and fitness problems. When the hips get out of alignment, virtually every joint in the body is affected.

After practicing this pose, in time the joints of the body will begin to realign back into the four-socket position that nature intended. This pose will increase functionality and begin to eliminate the pain from misaligned joints.

DIRECTIONS Lie on your back with one leg bent on a chair or block and the other leg extended on the floor. Make sure that your extended foot is propped against something *(Fig. 11.100)*. Simply relax and breathe fully and deeply with the diaphragm. In a short time, you'll begin to feel an easing of muscular tension. After you've spent time on one side, repeat and do the other leg.

Try to do an average of 10 to 15 minutes per side per session; even 5 minutes on each side will be of benefit. You can do up to 30 minutes per side. Because this pose is time consuming, I often recommend that people take 1 day a week off from their flexibility program and do the pose for 30 minutes to an hour per side. Although this may seem like a long time to do a pose, it will keep your hips relaxed for the entire week, thus eliminating having to do the stretch daily.

Fig. 11.100 Elevate one leg on a block and support the foot of the straight leg with a solid object

Alternate (S54A): Supine Groin Stretch—Elevated Leg

DIRECTIONS An even better way to do the supine groin stretch is to use a small stepladder, chair, bookcase, or multiple-position tower. Place your extended leg at an angle on a higher step or shelf and allow your foot to rest upon it. As your lower back relaxes into the floor, begin to lower your extended leg down to the next level until it finally rests on the floor. In other words, if you were to spend 20 minutes per side, start with your foot on the fourth rung of the stepladder and hold for 5 minutes. After 5 minutes, drop the leg down to the third rung and hold for 5 minutes, and so on. Or, using a chair, place your foot elevated on the seat of the chair for 10 minutes *(Fig. 11.100* on page 193) then down on the floor for 10 minutes.

Fig. 11.101 Elevate one leg on a chair or stepladder

S55. Supine Ball Roll

WARNING Do not do this stretch if you have back problems, especially disc involvement, as it puts stress on your lower back. As your back problems get better, begin to do this stretch under the supervision of a qualified person well versed in anatomical function.

BENEFIT This is a fabulous stretch to lengthen your entire body and especially your abdomen, chest, and shoulders.

DIRECTIONS You will need an exercise ball for this stretch. Lie on your back on the ball *(Fig. 11.102)*. Slowly roll back and forth, getting a nice massage of the back. Do this for 1 minute. This pose counters the solo sitting wall (S17, page 160) and further helps stretch the anterior muscle chains, while increasing stability in the posterior chains.

Fig. 11.102 Slowly roll back and forth, massaging the back

THE MIND-BODY CONNECTION

"Son, you don't have to be dumb to play good golf, but it really helps."
—JOHNNY REVOLTA, Member, PGA Hall of Fame

THAT PROFOUND STATEMENT was made to me by the late Johnny Revolta, who I still feel was one of the greatest teachers of all time, a man from whom I learned a tremendous amount. He said that to me after I asked him my usual myriad of technical questions about the golf swing. The reason for him saying this to me was an attempt to get me to stop thinking so much and start swinging by feel. I don't think many people would disagree with the statement that golf is the most mind-twisting and baffling sport ever devised by mankind, and it always amazes me what this game does to people, mentally and emotionally. In fact, one of the best things that happened to me and my psyche was becoming a golf instructor, because after some time, I realized I wasn't the only one that golf drove bananas!

Over all the years of teaching golf, I've literally seen grown, successful, and mature men completely lose their composure and throw and break clubs, curse hysterically, and yes—even break down and cry (I'm serious), and I'm sure that you have had your moments, too.

IS GOLF A GAME OF WHO HITS IT THE BEST, OR WHO MISSES IT THE BEST?

One of the questions that puzzles *every* golfer is why they have it one day and completely lose it the next? This even occurs from hole to hole—from shot to shot, from high handicappers to pros. Ben Hogan, arguably the greatest ball striker that ever lived, said that during an "exceptional" round of golf, he'd only hit around five or six shots that came off just how he wanted! In my way of understanding, that means he was hitting a *lot* of misses (in his case, a *lot* of good misses!). Since he's probably the greatest shot maker of all time, what does that say about the rest of us?

The emergence of sports and golf psychologists has played a substantial role in helping golfers focus, develop confidence, and control their emotions—all in an attempt to control their minds and eventually play better golf. No doubt about it, golf, like everything in life, is largely between the ears.

THE DIFFERENCE BETWEEN GREAT PLAYERS AND AMATEURS

I've been extremely blessed in having had the opportunity to have worked on the swings and bodies of many of the greatest players that have ever lived, not to mention Hall of Fame athletes from nearly every sport.

While working with and getting to know them, they've taken me into their confidence and shared with me many of their innermost feelings and insights regarding how they go about swinging the club and playing golf. Not only pro golfers, but the scores of great athletes from other sports have also offered their insights on how they approached and played their own sports.

One of the things I've noticed is that *all* of the pros have one thing in common: They all see things differently than us mortals, and they have an inner dialogue with themselves that is remarkably different from that of the amateurs. I've been asked thousands of times, "What are they like?" I've come to answer that question by saying, "Whatever you do, don't get in the way of a great champion and their target, because their eyes will burn a hole through you!" They also seem to have a special physiological gift of some sort, whether it's Arnold Palmer's shoulders, Chi Chi Rodriguez's hands, Jack Nicklaus's legs, and so forth.

Back to the visualizing. Palmer told me that he was fixated on the target and tried to "shake hands with it." I've heard Nicklaus say that at Augusta he felt he was in a "Fairyland type of environment" and got caught up in it—watching the breeze blow through the tops of the trees, the ripples in the pond, the flag blowing in response to the wind swirling around Amen Corner. I remember NFL Hall of Fame cornerback Mike Haynes describing to me how he would visualize the receiver he was going to cover in an upcoming Super Bowl and see himself intercepting a pass (which he actually did in the game). I've never met a great athlete in any sport who didn't visualize and see things in a way that's totally different from a high handicapper.

Along these lines, I remember reading about a case study once where a group of Tour players and amateurs were wired up to electroencephalogram machines while they performed their golf swings. Interestingly enough, the Tour players' brains were very quiet and didn't show much activity, whereas the higher handicapper brains were very active! Having taught thousands of golfers, there's no doubt that amateurs think too much. As where Tour players visualize their shots in their own way, I've found that most amateurs don't even aim, let alone visualize their shots. Then, during their swing, they're usually thinking about their mechanics rather than freeing their mind and allowing their natural instincts to take over and let it go.

In my view, this all boils down to anxiety and fear, or a lack of self-trust on the golfer's part; and it doesn't take a rocket scientist to understand that fear and anxiety will usually ruin a person's golf swing (or, really, just about any activity or situation on the planet). Relaxation and calmness are crucial in performing a golf swing, and if a golfer is thinking and worrying about whether or not he is in the right position, or thinking about this tip or that, then he is obviously trying to control the situation. Attempting to control a golf swing usually leads to overcontrol, which then inhibits your body from swinging freely. I've always loved what George Knudson, the Canadian professional and great ball striker, used to say, "To get control, you've got to give up control."

On the same topic, a reporter once asked Julius Boros what he would normally do when he came to a super-narrow fairway and had to hit it straight. Julius replied, "Baby, I just pour the coals to it."

"IT FEELS LIKE 'NOTHING'"

When great players or athletes are asked about what they were thinking when they were playing at the top of their game, they almost invariably reply that "things were very clear out there" or "everything seemed to 'slow down'—it seemed effortless." I remember listening to an interview with Jackie Stewart, the great race car driver, after he won the Indy 500. He said, "Everything seemed to be going in slow motion out there today." Think about it, here's a guy driving around 200 miles per hour in heavy traffic and he felt like it was all in slow motion. Again, nearly every athlete who's playing well—no matter the sport—understands this.

Any golf instructor will tell you that when they ask a student who has just hit a good shot during a lesson, "What did that feel like," the response is usually something like, "It felt like 'nothing.'" The bottom line is that when a person hits a good shot, he has pretty much cleared his mind; and when he hits a bad one, his mind is cluttered with thoughts.

The answer then is to clear your mind, and the question is: How do you do that?

WHAT'S GOING ON IN THERE?

The reality is that you've hit great shots many times before, and I can assure you that those good swings and good shots are still embedded deep in your brain. Unless you're a brand-new golfer, your body *knows* how to do it. Unfortunately, the bad shots and swings are embedded, too. The trick here is to be able to allow your mind/body to hit the shot via your swing without interruption from your conscious mind. Before I go any further, let's take a general look at how the brain and nervous system function.

While your eyes are looking at the target, your brain is collecting millions of bits of data and processing them in its magnificent computer. In essence, it's collecting data and sensory input that your conscious mind isn't even aware of. Once your brain has inputted the data, the brain's motor system is ready to send a signal out through the body via the nervous system and into your muscles.

One clear example is when you play catch with someone. Think about what a marvelous and ingenious action your brain does when you catch a ball. It sees the ball coming, then in a millisecond your brain figures out just where the ball will be in time and space, and it automatically puts your hand out there to catch it. I can assure you that you're not trying to figure out all the mechanics of your torso, hands, and arms in this natural and simple motion—but rather just doing it.

Again, this signal happens before you begin the motion. When the signal is uninterrupted and your body gets the message, you have some pretty good odds at making a good shot.

However, there's another aspect of the brain, called the prefrontal cortex, that deals with our thoughts, mediates conflicts, determines right and wrong, and so on. The problem here is that when the motor system sends the signal out to the body, it passes through the prefrontal cortex, which often interrupts the signal. When the signal is interrupted by the prefrontal cortex, the body doesn't get the message, in which case, the bigger and bulkier muscles begin to take over. In other words, your computer now has a bug in it and the programming from your brain to your body has been interrupted and short-circuited. Rather than performing the swing that the brain had originally programmed, you're now rolling the dice and hoping that the shot ends up good.

By now you're probably asking yourself, "What does all this have to do with flexibility?" The answer is *a lot!* As I've explained previously, a flexible muscle is just a relaxed muscle, and a relaxed muscle is one that gets oxygen, blood, and neurons to it. When the nerve spindles are relaxed and calm, the brain has a much easier time sending the signal out through the body and hitting the preprogrammed shot.

HOW TO NUMB YOUR MIND

One way to keep our bodies free from anxiety and excess is through breathing. Proper breathing, specifically east-west breathing (described in Chapter 10), is a great way to allow our bodies to be oxygenated and allow the signal from the brain to program the nerves and muscles throughout the body, and thus hit a good shot.

After taking a few breaths during your pre-shot routine, take your address position while occasionally looking at the target to visualize the shot you wish to hit. Now—right before you take the club back—allow your navel and lower diaphragm to expand outward. *Do this gently and keep it relaxed!* You can practice this by placing your right hand just under your belly button and gently pushing out on it. From here the club will tend to float back, and your relaxed muscles will allow your brain to send out the signals uninterrupted throughout your body and provide you with a much better chance to hit a good shot, which, *again*, your body knows how to do!

One thing that I cringe upon hearing is when an instructor advises a student to "tighten their core" and abs before and during their swing. Although having strong abs is a definite plus, when most people attempt to do this, they're inviting tension to creep into their

Fig. 12.1. Relaxing the lower diaphragm and *gently* pushing out ensures a smooth takeaway.

swing, and again, tension is the last thing we want. Tensing up will certainly retard your signal from programming your muscles.

AHHHHH-ING

Another excellent technique to shut off your mind is *Ahhhhh*-ing. I'm sure you're wondering what the heck that is. This is a technique that I learned from Ed Tischler, an excellent teacher whom I originally met in Hawaii.

Here's how it works: As you're addressing the ball, begin gently expelling your breath and literally say, "*Ahhhhh*" (just like what the doctor asks you to do when he examines your throat). If your mind is clear, you'll be able to

hold the same tone evenly throughout the entire swing. However, if you're tense or have some herky-jerky motions in your swing, you'll see that the *Ahhhhh* sound will be herky-jerky, too. We want the sound to be an even tone throughout your swing. This is an outstanding drill not only to calm your mind but also to create fluidity in your swing, as well as let the signal flow throughout your body.

DON'T LOOK BEHIND THAT CURTAIN

I attended a workshop in Florida conducted by Steven Yellin, who has come up with some excellent drills to empty and calm one's mind. One of the drills was called the surfboard drill, where after looking at the target during your preshot routine and address position, you imagine that a surfboard is standing straight up and placed in the middle of the ball. In other words, it blocks out the view of the target (which you've already programmed). Rather than use the surfboard as the obstruction, I prefer to visualize a curtain.

Here's how you do it: Stand behind the ball and visualize the shot you want while breathing softly. You've now programmed your motor system. After addressing the ball, take a few more peeks with your eyes—reinforcing your brain to send the signal throughout your body. Now draw an imaginary curtain that is about 10 feet high and just behind and outside of your left shoulder. Your target is now obstructed by the curtain. From here on out, don't look—or think—beyond the ball. Just swing with your mind numb. Although there's an old adage that says, "The ball is not the target, the target is the target"—which is obviously true—sometimes focusing on the target *too much*, can create anxiety and tension and actually block that signal.

These are only a few techniques that I've found effective, and like anything else, the more you practice shutting off your mind, the better you'll get at it.

And that's not too dumb of a thing to do!

WHAT TO EXPECT

NEARLY EVERY ONE of my clients asks me, "How long will it take before I see results?" Obviously, there is no one right answer, simply because everybody is different and comes from a different level of anatomical function. However, for the average person, there are some common trends.

Most people begin to see improvements in the first few days, mainly in that they're able to go further and deeper in the stretches, and the stretches become easier to do. It's exciting when they see themselves improving. In around 3 weeks, most people notice more and more freedom in their bodies and in their golf swings. As Arnold Palmer told me many times, "Something is happening to me. I feel lighter and taller." This brings up an interesting point. I've seen people regain up to 2 to 3 inches in height

after embarking on the program. Do they actually grow? Of course not. Rather, their muscles begin to elongate and come out of flexion. They begin to stand up straighter and taller because their tight muscles aren't pulling them forward in a rounded/hunchbacked posture.

The most noticeable improvement comes after 2 to 3 months, right around 90 days. Around this time, people's bodies and their golf swings begin to transform. Many of them literally have a glow about them and look more energetic and alive. The truth is they *are* more alive, simply because their bodies are more oxygenated. Their eyes actually have more sparkle. We are, after all, oxygen critters and desperately need oxygen to pervade our bodies. Depriving our bodies of oxygen for even a few minutes usually ends our life.

After 9 months, students who have consistently maintained their programs have become different people. Their entire anatomical function has changed, for the better.

If you're not experiencing improvements, then be honest with yourself. Are you doing the program consistently? Are you breathing deeply and fully? Are you doing enough of the programs? (Remember, this program only works *if* you work it!)

If you've answered yes to these questions, then maybe there are some other things going on. How's your diet? If you're eating too much meat (especially red) or junk food, your system will get clogged, which will prevent the oxygen and blood flow from effectively getting into the nerve spindle and nerve fibers.

Are you doing too much weight lifting or running? Although resistance training and cardiovascular training are crucial, too much of a good thing can sometimes be a bad thing. Get checked out by a knowledgeable physical trainer who is versed in anatomical function. You also might want to see a good nutritionist.

If the muscles are receiving oxygen and blood and you're working the muscle chains properly, your muscles must expand more deeply. If not, look at what else you may be doing that may be impeding your progress.

I cannot express enough the importance of having fun and keeping a positive attitude about your program. I want you to expect to improve and know that you're going to improve! A positive mind will produce positive results. I've seen a lot of people who had nothing wrong with them but didn't get results because of their negative attitudes. I have been incredibly fortunate to have gotten to know

and coach many of the greatest golfers, athletes, and business leaders, and I have yet to see one of them with a negative attitude. Not one! Those people are great because they set a goal and nothing is going to stop them. I want you to possess the same attitude. If you do, you'll be amazed before you're halfway through.

THE JACK NICKLAUS INSPIRATION STORY

When on this topic, I always feel compelled to share this true story about the greatest golfer who ever lived.

One day, Jack Nicklaus was in Pete Egoscue's clinic, and one of Pete's clients had his young son with him. Upon learning that Jack was in the clinic, the man asked Pete if his son could be introduced to Mr. Nicklaus and hopefully have Jack give him some words of wisdom.

As the introductions were made, Jack asked the boy what he liked to do. The boy responded that he loved to play golf and aspired to grow up and be a professional golfer "just like you, Mr. Nicklaus." Jack acknowledged him and then asked, "What else do you like to do, and what other sports do you play?" The boy replied that he really didn't play any other sports or do many other things, just golf.

Jack said, "Well, son, if that's the case, I would get off of that regimen of only playing golf and get out there and also try other sports and do as many other things as you can. I highly recommend that you not just play golf." He then added, "And before you go expand your life, remember that life is short, and the most important thing you can do for yourself is to stay fit. After all, you can have all the money, power, pride, and prestige in the world, but if you don't have your health, you're a poor man." He then followed up by sharing how he had been successful but was encumbered by several physical ailments, and now, because he was taking more responsibility for his health, he was feeling great again. "So, son, my final advice for you is to keep yourself fit."

The boy didn't look like he got the message, but I can assure you, the rest of us standing in that room that day sure did! Great advice from a great champion!

I want to close this book by saying that there was a long time in my life when I didn't take care of myself and, as a result, I lived in pain. It's been a long time since those days, and I can now say that I live pain-free. I say without hesitation that feeling good is what it's all about! And for me it starts with flexibility.

Speaking of feeling better, nothing makes me feel better than when I bump into people at the golf course, in restaurants, or wherever, and they stop me and share their positive testimonials of how these flexibility programs have changed their lives, improved their golf games, and changed their health for the better. I hope you get on these programs and see these results for yourself, and hopefully one day we can meet, so you, too, can make my day!

ACKNOWLEDGMENTS

I have a strong belief that all people are given certain gifts by the Creator, gifts that can manifest in an amazing variety of ways. I believe that if there is a secret to life, it just may be for each of us to discover what our individual gifts are and then use them, not only to help us go through life's many twists and turns, but especially to share them with others. I believe that one of the gifts that I've been given is the incredible number of fascinating people and friends—from all walks of life—that have come into and played a role in my life. Unfortunately, there are too many people that have influenced me to name here, but I would like to thank the ones who have contributed the most to the creation of this book.

I am especially grateful to David Chapman (my jockey) for believing in my message and putting together the amazing partnership that I have today. David, you are the man! To Charlie Mechem (the Godfather), whose wisdom, counsel, and especially friendship have helped me in more ways than I can express. To Arnold Palmer, for letting me hang out in his "kingdom" and allowing me to see his genius on how to treat people up close.

To Tommy Jacobs, whose friendship and belief in my message set the stage for this book. To Jim Achenbach, for hearing my message and using his professionalism to take the knowledge out of my head and onto these pages. To Ric McDonald and Pete Egoscue, for opening my eyes to a "functional world."

To my mother, Doris Fredericks, whose unshakable and positive personality was felt by all, and to my father, Elmer Fredericks, for teaching me to see the truth in all things.

To my wonderful and incredible wife, Jean, my lover and best friend, who always brings me back to seeing things clearly; and to my son, Ryan, for being the inspiration of my life.

And most of all, to the legions of people and students who have certainly taught me far more than I've ever taught them. I thank you all for giving me your gifts.

ESSENTIAL EQUIPMENT CHECKLIST

The following equipment will help you get the most from the drills and stretches prescribed in this book.

All available at FredericksGolf.com

Stretch rope, featured in supine leg chain
(S7, page 153)

Slant board, featured in standing drop-off
(with gluteal contractions) (S12, page 156)

Exercise ball, featured in Russian ball twist
(S34, page 175)

Power fan, featured in power fan drill
(D17, page 112)

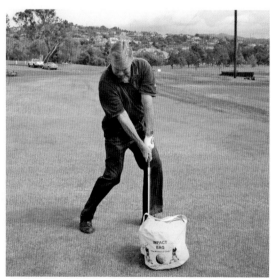

Impact bag, featured in impact bag drill
(D18, page 113)

ALSO FROM ROGER

Roger reveals more true secrets to the golf swing in his bestselling three-part DVD series, *Roger Fredericks Reveals Secrets to Golf Swing Flexibility*.

Featuring secrets to:

Secrets to Golf Swing Flexibility DVD

Secrets to a Fundamental Golf Swing DVD

Secrets to a Powerful Golf Swing DVD

Continuing Education Series #1: *Roger Fredericks Reveals Secrets to Longer Drives* DVD

Continuing Education Series #2: *Roger Fredericks Reveals Secrets to the Short Game* vol. 1: *Putting and Chipping* DVD

Continuing Education Series #3: *Roger Fredericks Reveals Secrets to the Short Game* vol. 2: *Wedges around the Green* DVD

Continuing Education Series #4: *Roger Fredericks Reveals Secrets: Flexible Solutions to Inflexible Swing Faults* DVD

All available at FredericksGolf.com

About the Author

For more than 20 years, Roger Fredericks has been one of the most influential and true pioneers of the golf fitness movement as well as one of the few golf professionals who is an expert in both golf instruction and in physiology. Roger has worked on the golf swings and bodies of more than 20,000 golfers, including more than 60 tour professionals and seven hall of famers. The creator of the smash hit infomercial "Roger Fredericks Reveals Secrets to Golf Swing Flexibility," he frequently travels around the country conducting golf outings, seminars, and speaking engagements. Roger resides in San Diego, California, where he offers his Golf Instruction and Flexibility Programs.

INDEX

Boldface page references indicate illustrations/photographs.